THIS LIFE WAS NEVER IN THE BROCHURE

Caring for Our Son With Severe Autism and Profound Multiple Learning Disabilities

---

NADINE HONEYBONE

authors
AND CO.

Medical Disclaimer

This book contains general information about medications and treatments. The information is not advice, and should not be treated as such. Do not substitute this information for the medical advice of physicians. The information contained in this book is based on the personal and professional experiences of the author. Always consult your doctor for yours' and your family's individual needs.

Dedication

My love, my life, my everything, and this book, is dedicated to my son, Tommy.

Throughout it all, you have my unconditional love, and I know I have yours too.

Praise for Nadine Honeybone

There are not many times I use the word inspirational, but that's exactly what Nadine is.

Nadine was one of the first people I met when I first started my journey on the ASD rollercoaster. She was the first person I talked to who got it. She validated my feelings and gave me hope. I was at my lowest point, I felt so alone, and Nadine very quickly and very effortlessly made me feel part of a group, actually, it was more than that, we were part of a family. When a lot of people would flounder, she set about helping others, using what little time she had to support other families and creating the Autism Directory, and now Autistic Minds. She showed me that an autism diagnosis wasn't the end of the world I felt it was. I am forever grateful. Nadine, don't you ever doubt the power of your reach.

Jo Paskell

Acknowledgements

With Huge Thanks to:

Tommy. You have rocked my world and I am so proud to be your mum. Love you lots like Jelly Tots.

Alun. You have loved, supported and stayed with me through it all. Jelly xxx.

Meg, Simon and Otis. You will never know how grateful we are to have you in our lives. Thank you, for all you have done for the three of us - and to Otis for your very special therapy cuddles. We are so honoured and proud to be part of your family and for you to be part of ours.

Ysgol-Y-Deri. The support you have given us all as a family has been phenomenal. We are so very grateful. Thank you.

Debra, Sarah and Suzanne and all his personal assistants over the years. Thank you for your support of Tommy and your care for him.

David. You came to us as a cleaner, but you've done everything around the house to keep it and us still functioning. You are part of our family too. Thank you.

Friends and Family. Thank you for your support throughout our journey. It takes a village they say. It certainly does.

Contents

Preface

This Life Was Never in the Brochure

Who knows what the journey will be like when you decide to start a family? It would not be unreasonable to think that it will be like many other journeys of parents you know, with some differences of course. But the typical journey through the early years of school, friends, holidays, teenage challenges, exams, partners, first car, further education and getting a job would be what you would generally expect.

But what if the parenting manual you reach out for, and there are thousands out there for all kinds of approaches and challenges to raising your children, doesn't actually touch on anything like the life you are actually living with your child?

Raising a child with severe autism and profound multiple learning disabilities (PMLD) is not a typical parenting journey and nothing you read in any of these parenting manuals has any relevance to your situation, your child or your challenges. We found them so annoying with their assumptions of when and what your child should be capable of that it really hurt to read them.

Our son, Tommy, was born in 2004 and received a diagnosis of autism when he was two years old. We were told lots of things such as he would "develop in his own time", told that "autism is really a gift", and that with therapies he could "lead a normal life". Eighteen years on and none of that ever came true. Tommy is an adult child. Physically, he is a man that wouldn't look out of place in the front row of a rugby scrum; a natural-born tight-head prop. Tall and very strong but developmentally still a toddler with limited capacity to understand and process the world around him, unable to make decisions for himself. Tommy also has a limited capacity to process his emotions and anxieties. Non-verbal, unable to communicate basic wants and needs, unable to say if he is hurting or scared, Tommy uses physical aggression to vent his frustration of not being heard and relies on carers to do absolutely everything for him.

Our parenting journey started with the visions and dreams that I saw in my imagination, taken from the perfect 'Brochure' of how to start and grow a family. The Brochure that sells you on the ideal life and joys of having children. For me, my vision was raising a child that goes on to do wonderful things, the great holidays we will go on, the school and exam successes. Everything from riding their first bike to buying them their first car, the friends and relationships they will have, growing up, being independent and being proud of whom they have become with their parents' guidance and love.

Our actual parenting journey was never in any Brochure. As we came across challenge after challenge we would find ourselves regularly saying to each other, "This was never in the Brochure."

This is our journey of raising our son Tommy. A child, and now an adult with severe autism and profound multiple learning disabilities.

Ours has not been a typical journey. But it is not an uncommon journey for many thousands of parents across the world who are experiencing the same things, day in and day out, as we have experienced. There are no manuals for this journey and certainly no

Brochures you would want to pick up to choose such a journey.

We have been to hell and back. But on days when we didn't honestly think we could get through another hour - we did. I have pulled myself out of traumatic stress to now believe in a good and happy future for Tommy and ourselves. Some of it was knowing how to get the practical resources needed. Most of it was about knowing where I was emotionally and the internal resources needed to travel this path and come out of it with my mental well-being intact.

This book is about our journey; the three of us. So far.

About the Author

I'm a mother to one very special child, Tommy, whom I had when I was forty after many struggles with conceiving and on our third IVF attempt. I am also a wife to Alun, who has journeyed with me and is thankfully still my husband.

My motherhood journey has not been typical. Tommy lost all development at fifteen months and had an early diagnosis of autism at two, followed by a learning disability. After the diagnosis, I went online and researched. I found a website near the top of the search list which said I needed to buy this product from America to help cure him. Who was I to know what was true and what was misinformation? I learnt the hard way about what's out there to help and guide parents in their journey with autism.

I connected with other parents who told me, "There is no help at all" but I looked and found some and started putting them on a spreadsheet which grew quite large. I then decided to share my research and launched *The Autism Directory* in September 2010 which became a registered charity in September 2011. It's now quite an organisation and after a name change, I continue to be the CEO of the award-winning charity, *Autistic Minds*.

In my career, I have also qualified as a Professional Coach, Master NLP Practitioner, Coach of Broadband Consciousness and delivered many life coaching sessions and programmes. I also consider myself to be a 'Master Manifester'. I have won awards from 'Coach of the Year' in 2010, 'Inspiring Woman in the Community' in 2012, 'Specialist Coach of the Year' in 2013. Then in 2019 a 'Life Achievement' award. I was only fifty-five at the time and remember saying in my acceptance "Thank you but I haven't finished just yet. There is so much more to do". The skills I gained through this work have helped me so much in this parenting journey, but none of it prepared me for the darkest days of my life.

From 2020 through 2022 were dark days and I was diagnosed with Traumatic Stress Disorder, Depression and Sleep Deprivation. I was completely broken by the care system and the life we had. I had hit rock bottom a few times in those years yet managed to keep going. In October 2021 I went so deep that I knew I had to make some decisions about my life if I was going to survive. I eventually found a small light of hope to cling onto and eventually got back to finding myself again.

Finding Me Again - Who Am I?

I am late fifties (at the time of writing obviously), and I wear my heart on my sleeve. You know what mood I am in because I can't fake it. I am an introvert pretending to be an extrovert, I love my own company but I like to party too as long as there aren't big crowds.

I have a need for the feeling of achievement and whatever I do needs to have a purpose; whether work, family or social. I am grateful for all the things I achieve each day, the main one being waking up in the morning.

I am trusting of people, I believe they will do things if they say they will (because I do that), and I want to see the best in others and give/receive lots of love and hugs.

A recovering self-critic who once had very little confidence and doubted herself, especially when challenged by others with a different point of view.

A recovering perfectionist who now understands that life is messy, and if you want to live life to the full then you accept it all – the good, the bad and the lessons learnt. On that note, I believe that being vulnerable is a great strength.

A recovering rescuer and fixer who wants nothing more than to help others heal, but also know that when I stop trying to rescue or fix and just love and be present, then their healing can begin.

That's the main reason I wrote this book. To help you heal. While you read it please know I hear you, I love you and I am present with you through your own healing.

ONE

Happy Ever After

I didn't need the alarm to wake me this morning. The car is ready and just needs the last few items to be packed and we can get going. I don't take the kitchen sink any more, but I still pack probably far too many shoes and clothes.

We are not going far, just an hour or so west to the cottages in Carmarthenshire we have hired for the past four years. This is where Tommy knows and is able to settle quickly on our annual holiday with him. Each year he goes into the familiar cottage first and he gets to choose his bedroom. Every year so far he has chosen the middle one with the high double bed. I wonder if he will choose it again.

A lot has changed for him and us this last year. He has turned eighteen and is now seen as an adult. Decisions about his care and welfare are no longer just mine to make, I am part of a team that decides what is in his 'best interests'. That term made me shudder a few years ago when I first heard it from the social worker. Before eighteen I made all the decisions on his behalf as I knew him the best as his mother, however, now we have what's known as multidisciplinary team (MDT) meetings. These are with adult social services, medical professionals, school staff, mental health professionals, the courts and any therapists involved in his care to decide what is in his 'best interests' regarding where he lives and what care he receives. To me that term just meant they had the ability to take over and do what they think was right for him, or in my view, what was the cheapest for them.

It's still quite early in the morning and we won't be setting off for a while yet, so I go through my packing list and make sure we have all we need, then I will walk through the house room by room and see if there is anything else I think we will need and chuck that in the car too.

Tommy moved into a residential home three months after he was eighteen. The most difficult decision of my life was in trusting others to love him and care for him as I would. So for this year's holiday, his luggage will be packed by his care team and we will meet them at the cottage later. I have his box of slinkies packed which he will expect when we see him, and I keep checking that they are definitely packed as he will expect them, as he always has. Managing his expectations is one of the important things we have learnt he constantly needs. Each morning I used to tell him whether today was a school day or a play day, and who he was going to be with. I then got a sense from his reaction whether that was something he was pleased about or not.

Tommy has been pretty much non-verbal all his life. He learnt certain words and phrases that he knows will get him things, but he didn't always use them in the right context. He got really frustrated and angry if he wanted a slinky but got toast, as that is what he asked for. But to him it was just a word to be used to get something; a prompt to action for us. Often, he would say as many words as he could in the hope one was right.

At the age of around fifteen months old, we noticed that he had lost some of the words he had gained. He is a fan of Bob the Builder and this was something he used to say over and over again until he stopped. His behaviour changed too; pacing in the garden, upset and starting to bang his head. Concerned I took him to see the GP who referred us to CAMHS (Child and Adolescent Mental Health Services), who within fifteen minutes of his first appointment diagnosed him with autism. That was seventeen years ago and little did we realise how much our lives changed completely that day.

My husband Alun worked in London at the time and so once I'd left the clinic we had one of those, "Are you sitting down?" phone calls. However, neither of us knew anything about autism anyway so we were completely confused as to what to feel. We did feel it wasn't good though.

Back to preparing for our annual holiday. Looking at the clock it was almost time to leave. I called the carers and checked that all was okay at their end. They had told him that today he was going on holiday and showed him the pictures of the cottage that he knows so well. He had smiled. That made me happy to know as so much has changed for him this last year that keeping some normality and routine in his life was key to making this work. They couldn't have told him much earlier than this morning as he lives pretty much in the present and would have expected to get in the car and go straight away.

I was so looking forward to seeing him again, and now I knew he was in a good place I relaxed and finished our final preparations. Alun and I then got in the car to set off west to meet our son; for the first time since he had moved out, I felt a huge relief and peace about going on holiday with him with no expectations of challenges and meltdowns that we would have to manage. That is now the responsibility of his carers and for once I can just be his mum, not his carer too.

The past eighteen years have been the most challenging of my life. I have felt feelings so profound and terrifyingly real; from depression and being completely broken, to elated feelings of unconditional love that I know I wouldn't have experienced without him in my life. And everything in between.

I fully expected parenting to be challenging at times and I knew from family and friends that had started that journey before me that it wasn't all fun, full of laughs and adventures. I did however have a vision in my mind about the parenting years, but what we experienced was never in the Brochure.

When we make the decision to start a family, we don't do it because of challenges and struggles we may face; But because of all the good things about being parents; a family, the joy and pride we will feel as we nurture and guide our children to become great human beings. The excitement of first steps, first words all the way up to exam results, their first car, relationships and where the journey may take them onwards, based on the foundations of love that we have given them. That's what's in the Brochure. That's what we expected.

Over the past eighteen years the phrase 'This was never in the Brochure' became a standard response from myself and Alun when we were truly challenged time after time with parenting a son with severe autism, profound multiple learning disability, a sensory processing disorder and more recently a mood disorder. The physical hurt, the trauma, the extreme emotional roller coaster, the desperation, the unconditional love, the deep reserves of patience and calmness that were needed at highly escalated times. The incredible strains that this puts on a couple were unprecedented.

This is *our* story. My desire for parents going through a similar journey is that our story gives you some hope, some help; support and some strategies to lead you to a happier self regardless of how your day has played out. I also want to help parents to develop faith in their own ability to still thrive and survive as an individual, to develop inner strength and to be okay with being vulnerable and being real.

I know how it feels to plummet into the depths of despair and not know what else to do; to not know how this will all end, to not know how to cope and how the hell to carry on. It has felt like I am drowning with no one there to throw me a lifebuoy; that my focus is just on surviving and getting through each day; on just keeping my head above water (and often going under) and on just making it to bedtime again.

That said; my own journey led me to be optimistic for the future and be able to handle daily life and its challenges much better. It led to my learning to trust and relinquish control of it all; to smile and laugh more; to re-establish better relationships with people around me and even love life again.

For anyone with a different story but still going through difficult times; I hope my own journey of raising consciousness through the challenges, of having hope through the despair, will inspire you. I will share the tools and strategies that I used to develop myself beyond what I thought was possible.

You never know how far you can go from the point where you thought it was the end.

"On particularly rough days when I'm sure I can't possibly endure, I like to remind myself that my track record for getting through bad days so far is 100%"

Author unknown

TWO

What's His Special Gift?

Reading about parenting and living with severe autism and profound multiple learning disabilities can be tough. It's a subject that isn't covered in general media and certainly not often portrayed in TV programmes, films or documentaries. Certainly, autism is being seen more and more now in soaps, dramas and films. But not the autism I know and have lived with every day for eighteen years. In 2018 there was a BBC TV Series *There She Goes* - a story about a young daughter with a learning disability, which has been the closest I've seen to depicting anything like our lives. However, even that wasn't close to our experience.

Not having any reference points like a film or drama that truly represents the life that both our son and us as parents are living, is difficult in many ways. The go-to film when you mention autism is *Rain Man,* which is so far from our reality that it makes it much more difficult to have a conversation with someone about how it's not like that at all or begin to try and change their perception of what others believe it is. Most people usually know someone with autism. Maybe a nephew, a friend's granddaughter, or a person at work who has a relative; this then becomes their view of what is meant by autism. Any deviation from that is challenging their own view and belief system, which to be honest, is generally not worth trying too. By the way, Kim Peek, the man upon whom the film Rain Man was based was not autistic. He had a learning disability and FG Syndrome.

The ignorance of others and the stupid questions they ask. Yes, it's understandable but still annoying. "What's his special gift? I've heard they have special gifts don't they?" Really? That question again? I've given many replies to that from "smearing poo wall art" to "slinky throwing" to "opening car doors on the motorway" and "throwing his slippers onto next-door's roof". Generally, though it's a more 'can't-be-bothered' reply such as "not all of them do" and walking away.

On more emotionally stronger days I can smile and remember that I once knew absolutely nothing about autism. I had heard the word but really had not come across any reference to autism with anyone I knew, anything I had seen nor even a conversation about it.

Early Years

Tommy was conceived with the help of IVF. Our third and final try after a naturally conceived miscarriage and two miscarriages from previous IVF attempts. We were living in London at the time and got to know the Lister Hospital very well over a few years. Different from my experiences of hospitals at the time, as it involved very steep invoices and the presentation of a credit card whenever we left or bought the drugs we needed. I'm pleased the NHS is now offering IVF to those who have difficulty conceiving as we did.

Before he was born we moved back home to South Wales to be closer to family and for him to be born Welsh - of course. Due to previous operations for endometriosis, it was a planned caesarean. It was booked for a Monday morning and we decided to tell no one. We just wanted some space for ourselves and for a few hours after he was delivered we just stayed with him; committed our unconditional love for him and stayed in the present with him, as a family, without distractions.

He was perfect. Still is. He was our whole world and stole our hearts which we willingly gave.

He grew and developed without any major concerns. He slept with me in my bed as he wouldn't settle in his basket or cot, he just wanted to be held and to be honest, all I wanted to do was to hold him too. All his milestones were met in terms of growth, weaning, crawling and walking.

When he was around fifteen months old we started to notice some changes, most noticeably was that the words he was learning and saying were no longer to be heard. Bob the Builder was one of the things he said a lot and all of a sudden he stopped saying it. We just hoped it was a phase and his talking would return. But the words didn't come back and never have. Our GP referred us to CAMHS (Child and Adolescent Mental Health Service) and at the first appointment, within fifteen minutes, Tommy had the diagnosis of autism.

Stunned and shocked we came away with our world in pieces. We didn't even know what autism was; but as it had been given as a diagnosis in a medical setting, by a doctor who looked sad when he told us, we assumed it was bad. Our world changed that day and set us on a path that has given us the biggest challenges in our lives, also the greatest learnings and self-discovery.

The first thing was to get on the internet to find out what this autism thing was and what I needed to do to help his recovery. I wasn't going to let this thing get in the way of the life I had dreamt of. I was determined to fix it. In my naivety at the time I thought this was a disease to be cured. I didn't know any better. It was after all a diagnosis from a medical professional and I knew of no other diagnosis that meant it was anything other than bad news.

The first thing I found out from my internet searches was that we needed to get a supplement called Glutathione but not just any one, it needed to be in a liquid format in order for it to be absorbed properly. It appeared that autism was due to a leaky gut which impacted the brain. So I believed at the time.

I have to caveat this by saying that I now know so much more about autism and work with some of the most amazing colleagues that have that diagnosis. I no longer believe that autism is something to be cured. I also believe that it's the comorbidities that often come with autism are the things that can make the presentation of autism so different, so much so that my son can be considered as having the same diagnosis as someone else who is highly skilled and intelligent.

What Is Autism?

"Autism is a lifelong developmental disability which affects how people communicate and interact with the world. More than one in 100 people are on the autism spectrum and there are around 700,000 autistic adults and children in the UK" - as defined by the National Autistic Society.

It is described as being a 'spectrum' which means that there is not just one way of seeing autism as everyone is different. There is a saying that "When you've met one person with autism, you've met ONE person with autism". However, I believe the linear way of how the spectrum is depicted, as in a horizontal line, is a bit outdated. It was meant to show where on the spectrum (line) someone is - with the left being 'high-functioning' or Asperger's and the right being more 'low-functioning' and needing more support. Firstly, describing someone as high or low functioning is derogatory. Secondly, what are the criteria for being at any point on the line, and thirdly, the challenges that are encountered are all different and cannot be ranked as more or less important than others.

Sensory challenges, anxiety, difficulties with executive functioning, communicating and social interaction are all things that can make life difficult to a greater or lesser degree. I saw a different approach to describe the spectrum which used a wheel – this showed on each spoke of the wheel a challenge that someone has due to their autism. The degree to which it was a challenge was depicted by where on the spoke they rated themselves; such as towards the centre of the wheel or towards the rim. This seems far more understandable and a better way to represent the spectrum. Each person has a unique representation and it's not higher or lower, better or worse than anyone else's.

Disability or Difference?

Is it a disability or a difference? I really don't know why there has to be such division in the autism community around this and so many other things that are not agreed on. My take on it is that a part of autism is seeing only one perspective, hence having difficulties seeing things from another person's point of view. That would go some way to understanding why there is such division in a community that shares a diagnosis.

Is it a disability? If someone feels disabled by their autism which limits them in life activities, then yes it is a disability for that person. The neurodiversity of autism also means it is a difference in the way the brain can interpret information, which isn't a disability but just a different way of thinking. For me it can be either or both.

A Gift?

Is it a gift? Oh wow, this one really stumped me in the beginning. There were challenges with Tommy, no doubt, but could his autism be seen as a gift? Many people do believe so and I would agree with them when talking about some of the brilliant autistic artists, musicians and IT geniuses I know who most definitely have a gift that their autism can amplify. Sharing a diagnosis with these people really shows how very different autistic people are, but so far, I couldn't find a gift in that sense.

Looking at the broader definition of a gift which we have learned to appreciate and understand is that he never, ever, displays an unearned emotion. He is incapable of emotional dishonesty. Every emotion he feels is writ large in his demeanour; be that boredom, neutrality, frustration, blissful elation, tiredness, unmitigated rage, contentment or hunger. While Tommy's expression of rage, frustration and anxiety can often be explosively destructive and violent, we know that he will not dwell on this. Within minutes after a violent and upsetting episode, Tommy will move on, put it behind him and be cheekily asking for toast with his trademark giggle. How he does this, we don't know, but what is clear is that he himself has developed internal strategies and tools for managing and processing his anxiety; we are grateful for that. All we have learned to do, when he has a meltdown, is to give him the space he needs.

This aspect of parenting Tommy has always been incredibly counter-intuitive. Our instinct, upon seeing a loved one in distress (and also self-harming in Tommy's case) is always to offer physical comfort and support. We gradually learned that this would never work with Tommy and would in fact exacerbate the situation. Many the time we have stood out of sight in the hallway near his bedroom, the sounds and noises indicating that he is having a bad time of it. But we both knew that intervention would just prolong things and we both knew that however painful it is to stand there giving Tommy his space, it won't be long before his own systems and strategies have kicked in and he will bring himself back to baseline and wander to the fridge, normally totally naked, and help himself to some grapes as if nothing had ever happened.

As a couple, we have learned so much from him about how to deal with and move on from conflict. We are a married couple within a highly pressurised, stressful, and often traumatic parenting infrastructure. We can bicker and squabble, sometimes over minutiae. That said, we seem to have each implicitly taken on Tommy's technique in that we never, ever dwell on any argument or conflict. It has been an incredibly healthy aspect of our journey, and a gift if we can call it that.

Autism or Autistic?

When referring to him should I be saying 'Tommy has autism' or 'Tommy is autistic'? I understand both viewpoints and I believe it's down to how someone sees their identity or the way in which they would like to be referred. I will always go along with their preference on this as it is about them and how they see themselves. It would not be polite, even rude, to refer to someone as 'she' when they see their own identity as 'he' or 'they'. I'm so pleased society is waking up to this from a gender perspective.

For me, the same goes for someone who identifies as autistic. What I mean by that is their autism is the core of who they are and their beliefs, values and behaviours are driven from that identity. The alternative is someone who has the diagnosis of autism but doesn't see it as something that drives all they do. Yes, they have autism which isn't separated from them; they may also have blonde hair, be short, wear glasses or a thousand other things that makeup who they are.

The stereotypes and societal norms we use to describe others with something different about them do not help in this context but by calling them out, they kind of do.

Talking of stereotypes, if you were to call someone blonde, rather than someone with blonde hair, it delivers a certain picture in one's mind about that person. In my era (it may be different now) but being referred to as blonde meant being a bit forgetful or ditzy. I had blonde hair when I was young and always used to say, "I have blonde hair but I am not blonde." It also became a thing to say "having a blonde moment" when describing something done that was a bit forgetful or dumb.

This is identity – word(s) that describe a bigger picture of someone, rather than a part or characteristic. The risk here is that stereotyping an autistic person means that people will get different views depending on the person they know as autistic, but apply that understanding to all Autistics.

Regarding societal norms, an argument I've heard is that 'you wouldn't refer to someone who is blind as they have blindness'. Probably not. That's only because we've learnt as a society to refer to them with the identity of 'blind'. They may not wish that identity and prefer to see it as one of many characteristics that they have, rather than it defining them as to who they only are. Also using 'with sight loss' is becoming a more useful description for those who do not want a blind identity.

Treatments and Therapies

The use of treatments and therapies is another contentious issue among the autistic and autism community (I use both terms now to include all, however they identify). When talking about a treatment it is often viewed as something to cure or reduce autism and that means some non-acceptance of the person as they are. It's akin to attempting to change or cure someone's personality just because it is different to the neurotypical view. If you just think of autism as being a different way of seeing the world around you, then I wholeheartedly agree that the neurodiversity of autism is about being and thinking differently and that brings a welcome difference to society as a whole. There is nothing here to be cured, except other people's view of neurodiversity.

However, the autism I know and what Tommy experiences is far from this. If there is a cure for being non-verbal or a treatment that prevents him from escalating into a meltdown and head banging to the point of cutting open his head, then I would be first in line. A therapy for helping him process and communicate pain is actually in his best interests; medication to calm sensory overload, or to help him sleep is his right to have. To me, treatments and therapies are just as important and helpful to the autistic and autism community as they are to all of society.

I mentioned before about the leaky gut, and whilst not the cause of autism I did find a connection between nutrition and his behaviours. Tommy was on a gluten and dairy free diet for a few years which made a noticeable difference in the beginning. Later on I found that sugar was contributing to his aggression and as soon as we reduced his intake, he become a lot calmer. Supplements were difficult to give him but using homeopathy was great for Tommy as he would take the little remedies and crunch them. He had a homeopathic first aid kit which really helped him with colds, digestion issues and other regular common ailments.

Tommy's Autism

Tommy's autism is unique to him. I describe it as severe autism because that's what it is. I'm aware there is a lot of controversy about labelling someone as 'severe' from the autism community itself but I really don't know why. I know many are proud of their autism and rightly so - if that's how they see it.

This is how Tommy's autism and his comorbid conditions have affected him since he was a baby to now, at eighteen.

- Apart from the occasional words that he knows gets him something he wants like biscuit or crisps, he is non-verbal. However, he doesn't relate the word crisps to a bag of crisps, or biscuit to a biscuit. He just knows that it's a word that gets him something he wants, which could be crisps, a biscuit, a drink, a slinky toy or anything really. It is just a prompt to action for those around him. For a while, Tommy used the word "water" almost exclusively when he wanted to communicate an idea about something he needed - whatever that was.

- He lacks the ability to use a communication tool to ask for something. We tried a few different ones but he got really frustrated and again could not relate what he wanted with a picture. As a baby, we started with PECS (Picture Exchange Communication System) whereby he thought that if he gave someone a picture card he would get what he wanted – whether that was the picture on the card or not. All this taught him was that the action of giving a picture card got him something; he didn't relate to the fact that the picture on the card had anything to do with it.

- He does communicate by taking your hand somewhere where there is something he wants. After a time you can figure out what this could be. If he took me to the larder he probably wanted something to eat; so I would get things down off the shelf one after the other until he stopped pushing them away as he finally got what he wanted. Or not. Taking me to the door meant he wanted to go to the car. Taking me to the bottom of the stairs meant he wanted me to go and get him a slinky toy. There were many times when he took me somewhere and I had no clue what he was after. This method generally worked well in the house and with people who knew what these things meant - but out in the community, it was so much more difficult.

- He has complex sensory needs. There is an optimum 'calm alert state' that he needs to be able to function and learn. Most of the time he is either below this and needs stimulation, or too high above this when he is hyper and needs bringing down. He has learnt over the years how to regulate himself by using the trampoline or with slinky toys. We often also have to help him with deep pressure or squeezes (strong hugs). When neither he nor we succeed in this he starts to escalate quickly which turns into a 'meltdown'. By meltdown, I don't mean a 'temper tantrum'. The difference is that a meltdown is completely uncontrollable and he can't just decide to stop it. Like an explosion. This is the hardest thing to watch as you feel completely helpless. He bites his fingers so hard and bangs his fists down on hard surfaces such as concrete or the marble worktop. He comes in for a squeeze to try and help himself but he then hits out with thumps and scratching. This is an uncontrollable behaviour as he just cannot process what is going for him in his mind and body. In later years this turned into headbanging the walls so hard that he left head-shaped dents in the plasterboard, or in extreme times he used concrete walls. All you can do is let him be alone, watch from a distance to ensure he stays safe, and then be there afterwards for him when he gets upset. This is heartbreaking.

- He lacks the cognitive ability to communicate that he is in pain. I've never known if he's had a headache; tummy ache, muscle pain or toothache as he is unable to process pain like we do and he cannot show or even point to any pain he has. This is so difficult to deal with especially when you know something isn't right. It's a basic human need to communicate pain and to indicate at least where. This alone upsets me so much.

- He is unaware of the concept of medicine or anything that could help; such as a cold towel, plaster or bandage. Anything you try gets pushed away or taken off and that's if you can even get near to him to administer anything. For example, one day he cut his foot in the house and he wouldn't let anyone near it. It was bleeding so while he sat on a kitchen bar stool the best I could do was to throw cups of water from a distance to attempt to wash and clean the wound. As for medication, like paracetamol or antibiotics, he would never take it. You can't even explain that it will make things better. If he didn't want to take it, he wouldn't. And he didn't. Not being able to help someone you love is painful. Seeing them suffer when you know you could help, but can't, is so tough.

- He also cannot process discomfort or pain. He never cried (apart from as a baby) and I have no idea how anything like a cut foot felt for him. If, when I dressed him, his pants were a bit skewwhiff or his t-shirt was not pulled down properly he wouldn't do anything. I don't know if that was because he didn't feel it or he just didn't know how to fix it for himself. One day he walked all day with a screw in his shoe that had fallen in before I put them on him.

- He cannot clean himself after going to the toilet. He cannot dress himself, although he is good at taking his clothes off. No concept of why he needs to wear clothes when he prefers not to at all – in or out of the house. Too often he would get his shoes to go out in the car and have nothing else on. He had developed the understanding that shoes were needed for the car, but not clothes.

- As an adult; Tommy is still a toddler. He watches *Bob the Builder* DVDs, uses his iPad for pre-school programmes, needs all his personal care done for him, needs his food prepared, clothes washed, hair washed, beard trimmed, nails cut, and every other need done for him too.

What I have found helpful is to learn what you actually think and believe. Don't get caught up on what you read on social media, what others think, and what others tell you to believe. If you are on all the socials you will find there are many people who will offer advice, or even tell you what to think. You, your partner, and your children are completely unique and if you start like we did knowing nothing about autism, that's okay. Be your own guide. Take advice, of course, but make your own decisions. Be willing to get things wrong. Have faith in your own ability to do this and accept it may be far from perfect. Be okay with that too.

I was so wrong about a lot of what I thought, but I was easily influenced, probably by fear and the need to fix things. As well as no Brochure, there is no guide map or manual. There can't be either. Learn to trust yourself and your instinct. By raising your consciousness you can get to a place where you know the journey is what it is and you don't have to resist or fight it. You will be given the opportunities you need and allowing yourself to be vulnerable will be your strength, your power. That will be your special gift.

THREE

Journey Into the Unknown

When we received the diagnosis of autism for Tommy we were flung into the deep end with no life jackets. Nothing was given to us, not even an information leaflet. We were just sent home after being told that this is a lifelong disability, there is no cure or medication to help.

I've mentioned before how my views have changed since that day, however, at the time it felt like a hopeless situation. Something had caused this in my beloved boy, but no one could tell me what. No one could tell me how to help him, what to do, who to speak to, and what this would mean for his life growing up.

Beyond Diagnosis

What I expected was that someone would be able to tell us what the next steps were and what to do. The National Autistic Society (NAS) seemed to be the people who would be able to explain all this to me, give me the information to start helping my boy and tell me how this is going to impact his life. They couldn't. I realise now that no one could have explained what was to come.

As he was only two the gap between the milestones he met and that of a typical two-year-old were hard to measure. The most distinctive gap was in his speech as he had lost the words he was previously saying, so we were referred to the speech and language team at the local children's hospital. But there was a waiting list. Eventually, we did have our first appointment. I can't recall exactly how long the wait was for it, but I think it was about a year which I was told was pretty good. I remember thinking at the time that it would be critical to start with speech therapy without hesitation if we were going to give him the best chance. How on earth can anyone think that a delay of around a year was pretty good? Especially at that age.

The problem is that we have normalised this expectation. Waiting for critical help and support across all health and social care services is now expected, therefore that's okay. We accept it. It's normal. We've been fed this line for so long that we think there is nothing we can do about it. We are constantly fed the narrative of a broken NHS with long wait queues so this has now become our norm. I'm not saying for one minute that this isn't the case, my point is that we've come to accept it because we've been told that's how it is. When it actually came to needing speech therapy to help Tommy do the most basic, and most important life skill that the majority of other children can do, it wasn't deemed urgent enough to not have to wait.

The inability to communicate needs, wants, pains, emotions, thoughts, questions, and troubles is just unthinkable. Yet that's what Tommy has lived with for eighteen years now. I don't know if a quicker start to speech therapy would have made any difference, but it certainly did not help avoid this incapacitating disability.

I started to learn more about autism. The first port of call was the internet; the initial websites and documents I read all described something called 'leaky gut' which affected the brain with toxins and the remedy was glutathione. After that episode of trying imported medication, not really knowing what I was doing or even what results I was expecting, I thought that there had to be other people in Wales and the UK that knew more and could help and advise. I started researching groups; training, organisations, and people of influence and then started to join in and mix with other parents whose children had the same diagnosis. I started to feel that we were not alone, and by chatting with others I also started to feel that this common diagnosis that our children shared was not consistent in its presentation. Other children were talking, out of nappies, off their bedtime milk, but not Tommy. In fact, we were finally (semi) successful in toilet training and stopped the nappies when he was eight, similarly with his milk. At the time I heard someone say that a friend's child hadn't started talking till he was twelve. That really derailed me. Is it possible that he wouldn't talk until he was twelve? That would be the worst thing I could imagine.

Education

I start to think about school and where he would go. Initially, we joined the local 'meithrin', a pre-nursery group in the local town for Welsh-speaking families. Although I don't speak Welsh, Alun does, and we were keen for Tommy to speak Welsh too. Of course, now I would give everything and anything for him to speak any bloody language and be able to communicate verbally.

When he was old enough for nursery (we had given up the idea of Welsh schooling) the nursery school for our area only took children that had been toilet trained. We had had his diagnosis by then so we had to figure out what was possible for him. That's when we had our first experience with children's social services and the constant testing, assessing and decisions being made for him began. He was assessed to need one-to-one support in the nursery to help with nappy changes and so was able to attend. No support to help him with the environment, noises or learning to play which were challenging for him, but someone to change his nappies. Nevertheless, we were thankful he could attend.

They really didn't have any experience with toddlers with autism. I don't know where the other children of his age with autism were, but he was the only one and it was a new experience for the staff. One day the alarm bells were set off and they had to evacuate the building. He became traumatised by the noise and they didn't know what to do with him or how to support him. After that day he displayed new behaviours in the nursery, throwing himself onto the floor, head banging the floor and walls with absolutely no awareness of what was in the way or what he would hit. This became increasingly challenging for them and I was often called in to pick him up.

The thought of him having to go to a special school was daunting. The only reference I had to special education was in my own comprehensive school which had a 'remedial' department and most of the children in there were segregated. Even in the late seventies, it should have been totally unacceptable to label children like this.

Thankfully we have a very special school near to us and although I had concerns when he started there, it turned out to be the best school ever. I will be forever grateful for their support for both Tommy and us - as a family - over the years he has been there. It was the subject of a BBC documentary series *A Very Special School* and called Ysgol Y Deri.

He needed a *Statement of Educational Needs*. A legal document which required an assessment so the most appropriate provision could be chosen for him.

Thankfully Ysgol Y Deri was stated as being the best to meet his needs by the local education authority. Not a decision we could make or even influence. If there are any positives at all for Tommy having severe autism is that we didn't have to fight like other parents often do for him to go to this amazing school.

That's pretty much the only fight we didn't have on our hands.

Social Services

As Tommy grew, the gap between his development and what was typical for his age also grew dramatically. With that came the challenges of sourcing things not meant for a child of his age. Nappies for an eight-year-old were not found in the local supermarkets. We found a service online to provide these but at a significant cost. After many requests, we eventually were successful (another assessment) for free specialist nappies delivered to the door. A provision that's available but no one knows or tells you about.

Tommy had multiple assessments each year and each time the gap was growing. His developmental abilities were not progressing at all. As he grew, the team around him grew, but not generally for his benefit. It was more of providing us with "help" that didn't provide any practical help at all. Just constant questions from different people and different teams asking me to relive the most challenging times with him over and over again. I would have to explain the sleepless nights as he didn't sleep long hours and getting him to bed was always a challenge. The anxiety started early in the morning as I woke with either a bang from him on his wall, or he would come into my room and I would see what behaviour he was displaying. Some mornings he was delightful and he would sit on my bed with his iPad. On other mornings it was aggression from the go and the first hit out or scratch to my arm was the start to my day. It was unpredictable.

I asked about some respite for us. It was getting to be that we just couldn't have any time to ourselves and each night was getting to be a challenge. Having a social worker didn't mean you could get what you needed. It just meant that if the social worker thought it was appropriate then they would mention it, but couldn't say whether it would be approved. That required an assessment, which would then go to the panel - a group of people in social services who don't know you or your child to decide whether to grant the thing you needed or not. It was never a quick process.

We were eventually awarded two nights a month of respite. This meant that Tommy would have an overnight stay at a local Action for Children centre, so we could have two nights of proper sleep a month from around the age of seven.

Statement of Educational Needs (SEN)

Being at a school for Special Education Needs meant that provision had to be reviewed each year and the 'statement of educational needs' would be re-assessed. Annually we would meet with social services and professionals involved in his education and therapies such as speech and language, occupational therapy and music therapy. While he was in the infant years at school he was being well supported by the interventions he needed, but each year the intensity and need for them were growing. However, whenever I asked for these needs to be acknowledged formally in his Statement, the Local Education Authority would always deny this.

The Statement is a legal document that describes the educational needs of the person and the provisions needed in order to access an educational curriculum. As a legal document whatever is in that Statement becomes an obligation for the local authority to provide. It was obvious why then that they refused to add these interventions into his Statement. Their argument was that he was receiving interventions so there was no need to include more. My argument was that by not being in the Statement they could easily take interventions away due to budget cuts or whatever else they could use to justify removing therapies needed. Tommy was coming to the end of his infant years at the school and about to start secondary. His needs were increasing and I feared they may not be able to provide the intensity of support he required.

The inclusion of these interventions in his Statement of Educational Needs was again denied by the Local Authority. I sought legal advice and began the process to take the Local Authority to a Tribunal Court in order to update his Statement to include the things he needed. I wasn't going to risk it. It was also a stand against The System that knew that if a parent contested anything the Local Authority did, they would have to use the Tribunal Process to resolve it. This was not an accessible route for many families as the cost of hiring an SEN solicitor was not cheap. The Local Authority knew this too.

This is not a fair system. I brought this up at a meeting of the Cross Party Autism Group at the Senedd (the

Welsh Parliament). In that discussion, they reiterated the fact that if there was any circumstance that the local authorities were not delivering on their contractual obligations (the Statement) then they had the legal system there to challenge it. My argument was that they absolutely knew that most families would not be able to afford this and were using this fact to bully parents into accepting a sub-standard, *Not Fit for Purpose*, Statement for their child. Another example of parents having no choice and feeling out of control with providing equality of opportunity to education access for their child.

I took the Local Authority to court and succeeded in having Tommy's Statement updated to include the interventions he needed; the frequency and length of time he would have these interventions and the professional level of staff that would work with him. The whole process took about a year and involved many independent assessments that we also had to pay for, plus the legal fees. The legal fees ran into the thousands but it was worth it to know he would get what he needed.

Therapies

His therapies in school included Occupational Therapy, Speech and Language Therapy and Music Therapy. Outside of school I also took him for Osteopathy.

It took me a while to get my head around his sensory needs, what a sensory diet was and why it was needed. He had a brilliant Occupational Therapist at school who really understood him and explained things to me - many times. As I understood it, which I still don't fully, is that the optimal place for him was in a 'calm-alert' place. So when he is lazing around and not engaging, with low movement, then sensory stimulation raises him to that middle ground where can start to access some kind of learning and development. However, it can often miss the middle ground and make him hyper. He is lovely when in this state for a short time as he runs about, laughs and is in a hyper mood, but it's not a good place for him to stay for too long. Sensory intervention was needed again to bring him down. However, he learnt to love it in this high place and would resist any efforts to lower his state. Initially, we experimented with weighted jackets and blankets, squeeze boxes and sensory rooms. It was all a bit hit and miss, but over time he began to regulate himself to increase or lower his state.

For most of us, we don't even have to think about sensory regulation. Our bodies deal with it and we automatically filter out certain noises or lower our sensory input from our environment. Background noise is just that. But what if every single noise around you was at the same level and you couldn't filter it out? Supermarkets are generally no-go areas; not just because of the noise levels of people and tannoys, but the change in temperature as you pass the fridges and freezers, the smell of the fish counter, bakery, or all the people moving around. Then there is the checkout before you can finally leave the place with the queuing and beeping. Imagine being constantly overwhelmed, every sensory dial on 'full input', with no easy way to regulate yourself.

Tommy loves his tight squeezes to this day and it's his favourite thing to do with people he knows. *Squeeze* is one of the few words Tommy knows how to use with its proper intent.

Medication

As he reached his mid-teens it was becoming more difficult to manage him and provide what he needed at home. My mental and physical health began to worsen dramatically. He was referred back to CAMHS and we had a psychiatrist appointment to begin the discussion of medication. I had heard a lot from other parents about this, whilst some views were positive about how it can help, others were against it in the belief that over-medicating to zombie them out wasn't good. I went in with an open mind to listen and understand what medication could do to help.

He was initially prescribed Fluoxetine. We had been through the issue of getting medication into him with the doctor, but we said we would have a go. The effect of the first dose had meant he refused any more – he could smell it, taste it in everything we tried to hide it in. After a short while with no success, we gave up. Knowing that this kind of medication needed to be regular we didn't have a choice. We tried to get back in touch with the psychiatrist but due to the pandemic, he was out of the country and couldn't return. We didn't get to speak to the psychiatrist for another two years.

Recently, now that Tommy has become an adult, he is able to be prescribed a wider range of medication. He has been prescribed Aripiprazole, Lorazepam as needed, and Sertraline. Fortunately, these don't seem to have taste issues and he takes them covertly in juice. They have really helped him and it has been so frustrating that he wasn't offered them before. Knowing what we now know about his anxiety, life in the past few years would have been so different for us all with this help. There doesn't seem to be any leeway for under eighteens having access to the medication that they need.

Health

In early 2020 his breath started to smell incredibly bad. We looked at trying to change elements of his diet but nothing seemed to change this. I was convinced that it was coming from his stomach and that something really bad was happening there. We met with a paediatrician at his school, as it was much easier to have appointments there than get him to the hospital. Somehow we managed to get a look up his nose, very briefly and saw there was something stuck at the top. I looked later and it was a small white mass at the very top of his left nose. We were asked to take him to the GP and get it removed.

I was not convinced it would be this easy. As soon as people seemed to get interested in seeing up his nose he wasn't having any of it. The GP asked a nurse to come in and they discussed something called a 'mothers kiss'. I was asked to hold his right nostril shut and blow into his mouth in an attempt to dislodge the foreign object. He found this hilarious but wouldn't let me close enough to do it. I could get close enough for a kiss but he wouldn't let me hold his nose, but he liked me blowing in his face.

So that wasn't a solution. The next step was to take him to the main children's hospital for an assessment. He wouldn't let anyone get close to have a look so the only option I was told was a general anaesthetic and a simple procedure. He had never had such an invasive procedure before and I was so concerned for him. With the help of Ysgol-Y-Deri school the planning was discussed with the hospital teams and a sensory room was provided for him to chill in before the procedure. The school also desensitised him to the gas mask by getting him to put it on his own face a number of times in school beforehand. When given the pre-med in a sweet drink he only took some of it, soon becoming wise that it was not just juice, however, it did make him quite relaxed.

I discovered from many times before that I am a complete mess in these situations with him. I think my own anxiety just doesn't help so the team from school was with him in the sensory room while I sat in a room next door. They went with him and helped them apply the mask which took effect very quickly thankfully. It wasn't a long procedure to get the object out of his nose and he was soon back in recovery. He still had the cannula in his hand and I asked the nurse to take it out before he woke but they said it was required in case they needed to administer any sickness medication. I knew what would happen when he did start to wake, the first thing he did was to try and pull it out. The nurse came quickly and removed it. He couldn't wait to get out of that room and tried to stand up. As soon as we could we got him home. I talked to him about it, but I really don't know what he understood. Times like these are excruciating when he can't express anything back to me, ask questions, or tell me how he is feeling.

A couple of months later the pandemic started; the worst time of my life was about to begin. His behaviour worsened and the meltdowns increased in frequency and severity. Meltdowns on the scale I had not seen before. I put it down to not being able to see his osteopath since the beginning of lockdown, something which he had been going to monthly. When he was due a session it was noticeable that he needed it. He really looked in pain at times. In these meltdowns he searched for a hard object he could get his teeth around and grabbed whatever he could to put in his mouth. Then he started on the doors, biting them on the sides, or he would get his teeth around the window sills where they jutted out. He bit down so hard on things I would notice the pain and fear in his eyes. One time he grabbed my hand which I tried to pull away. It was in a fist shape and he sunk his teeth right into my fingers and knuckles on the left-hand side. Painful doesn't do it justice. I ended up later in A&E concerned that the tendons had been damaged as I couldn't open my fist on that hand for a few days. I know he didn't mean to hurt me. I could tell by the way he looked at me he didn't want to hurt me but there was nothing else immediately available for him to bite on. It was excruciating pain but I know I couldn't scream out for fear of escalating him even further. I had learnt the best thing to do to support him was just look at him with love in my eyes and I did that this time too, without making a sound. I saw the large rope dog chew thing that we had bought recently and was able to get that and put it in his mouth to provide some relief.

These episodes continued to occur more frequently. I was constantly messaging social services and health teams for help. It wasn't an option for us to take him into A&E as we had no idea of the cause. He was in frequent pain without being able to tell me where. He doesn't have the capacity, or ability, to even point to it so we have always been in the dark, making assumptions about what could be wrong. Due to all the biting, my thoughts were definitely teeth related but all my attempts to get someone to help us just resulted in another MDT meeting to discuss but no action. I was getting more concerned and fearful every moment of every day over when the next meltdown was coming.

One evening when I could sense a meltdown coming, I went to comfort him the best way I could and he looked at me straight in the eyes and said, "Mummy." It would have been a wonderful moment if it wasn't for the fear I could see in his eyes and I knew he was asking for help. I was at a total loss over what to do. I held him close to reassure but I just didn't know what was wrong or what I could do. Even pain medication was so difficult to administer as he wouldn't take anything at all, not even Calpol. We had the idea to crush some paracetamol and mould it into some milky way which worked initially. He smells everything before putting it into his mouth and for the first few times he accepted the paracetamol chocolate until he became wise to it.

I called Social Services and Health again the next day, begging them to help me find out what was going on. I told them that I believed it was his teeth but he wouldn't let anyone look in his mouth, but he couldn't see a community dentist due to COVID. The team referred us to CAMHS for a virtual appointment as they thought the increased aggression could be anxiety related. The psychiatrist prescribed him with fluoxetine (also known as Prozac), an antidepressant. We gave this a try by disguising the liquid in juice, but each time he escalated soon after. I didn't think it was anxiety.

He began drinking water from the tap. He would put his face and mouth into the stream of cold water on a regular basis. Was this thirst an indication of diabetes? More calls to the team but no answers. To test would mean blood taken through a finger prick. He wouldn't allow this, forcing this on him through restraint was also a no-go. Every interaction with health had to be done in a manner that reinforced he was safe and okay, in order for him to develop that sense of being *okay* for the rest of his life when needing medical attention.

Many months, emails, call and emails passed. He was eventually referred to a dental hospital in Cardiff. We knew from previous experience with the Community Dentist that he wouldn't comply with opening his mouth for anyone to look inside. His school, Ysgol y Deri, were hugely supportive and they sent in a behaviour team of people he knew to the assessment appointment. I'm just a huge mess in these situations. All I can do is cry and I'm no good to anyone. The team were brilliant with him and although we knew he wouldn't open his mouth willingly, a biscuit provided them with enough of a glance to see a black space which warranted further investigation. This would only be possible under general anaesthetic. Again he needed a GA in the space of less than a year to perform a procedure for the simplest of things.

We had to wait two months. In the midst of the pandemic when only urgent cases were being seen it was a long wait, but thankfully he had a date at least. Meanwhile, the meltdowns and the traumatic stress on us all took hold. He had to isolate beforehand which meant the support that we had during this time was removed. This was in December 2020 and he was turning sixteen. The Children's Hospital that had taken good care of him earlier that year was in doubt due to his age. However, it turned out that as the referral was made before his sixteenth birthday so he was allowed to be treated there, again we had use of the sensory room beforehand.

This time he wouldn't take the pre-med. So he was wheeled up to the theatre fully awake and needed restraining while the gas and air took effect. I couldn't be with him as I was in bits in the waiting room. Again, another team from the school was able to come with us and, thankfully took control over the situation, saving me from the hard emotional stuff. I waited in a separate room.

It took ages before I was told that the procedure had finished and he was in recovery. A while later he was brought back to his room very dosed up. As he woke he was not good. I've never been good after GA either, always with a lot of sickness. Every sip of water had him throwing up blood. It looked horrific with blood spurting out of his mouth. We were told that a lot of dental work had been done and a lot of blood would have been swallowed.

So what did they find? What they found was that he
had three teeth down to the raw nerve. They extracted
those and a few they couldn't save and repaired others.
They had warned me previously that they had to be
quite brutal in their decisions about whether to
remove or repair his teeth due to the fact that he
would always need dental work done via GA and his
mouth hygiene wasn't the best. I had to sign a form to
give authority for them to take the decisions they
deemed necessary during the procedure.

His recovery was slow as he came around from the
anaesthetic. More sips of water and more blood
coming up from the stomach. When he was more
'with it' he kept trying to stand up but, he didn't have
the strength in his legs. He just wanted to get out of
there. We were given the okay to take him home so I
went to get a wheelchair and as soon as I said "home"
you couldn't get him in it fast enough. He recovered
well at home and although he slept well I didn't at all
that night.

After that time his meltdowns stopped for a while
until Spring 2021 when they began again. What was it
now? Was it his teeth again? Was it something else?
This time my calls to the teams resulted in quicker
action. I was adamant that he wouldn't be allowed to

suffer all those months again while people deliberated over what it could be, or what to do to rule other stuff out first. He got an appointment with the Community Dental Nurse, but he wouldn't even open his mouth, not even for a biscuit.

Where were we to go from here? Does he need a GA every time I can see he is in pain? How could that work for the rest of his life? Without being able to look they said it was probably an ulcer in his mouth. Was it? Who knows?

I'm often asked whether his severe autism or profound multiple learning disabilities means his life expectancy is shorter. Statistics have shown that it is, but, not because of the conditions. These in themselves do not have a medical reason for any different life span. The issue is with his inability to communicate, and that he may have a medical issue which goes untreated.

This is why the health system is so important for Tommy, that there are staff there who really understand him. We've had good and bad experiences at our local A&E. They work flat out I know, and I am forever grateful for what they do. They need more resources and it's really not acceptable to be okay with the way it is managed and funded.

In 2022 during a meltdown, Tommy accidentally smashed a glass vase. It shouldn't have been in his way but it was in a room that we generally kept him away from. He had stood in it but we were unsure if his foot was cut at all. His behaviour was escalating so a team from his class in school came to take to get it checked by the school nurses. Unaware of there being glass in his foot, he was back to A&E with the team who helped and supported the staff in the hospital. Still, he wouldn't be on his own for an X-ray, so the amazing school staff were with him, holding him as still as possible while the X-ray was done. Thankfully it was clear.

Not long after, Tommy had a bee sting on his face which flared up overnight. His face was swollen so much you couldn't see his left eye at all. Back to A&E which was very busy this time. A meltdown in the waiting room meant he was moved to a smaller room. Doctor after doctor came in to see him and many opinions were made but without being able to see in his eye they initially suggested keeping him in overnight on an antibiotic drip. I knew he wouldn't have the needle in his hand and if they did get it in he would pull it out. We were also hassled by other patients because Tommy was playing Moana on repeat on his iPad. In the end, he was prescribed antibiotics, which I knew he wouldn't take, asked to bring him back the next day to see the Consultant Ophthalmologist. It turned out okay in the end and the swelling eventually subsided. But the experience was heart-rending, upsetting and very traumatic. Again.

I have found that people really do want to help. They want to understand and there is an increase in training provided and awareness in schools and hospitals; with allocated staff who can be your point of contact. It is difficult for A&E staff due to the pressures they are under, but for patients that need extra help and support it is critical to have these resources available to provide a good outcome for everyone involved.

I am extremely hurt by the way Tommy was allowed to continue suffering with his pain. For someone that could communicate it would have been sorted quickly, but due to his disabilities, he was genuinely left to suffer. I'm sure that his anxiety now has something to do with the trauma experienced at that time.

It's easy to be angry, but at the situation, not the people. I have found that in most cases those that are trying to help and support us are doing the best they can with what resources they have, be that time, money or anything else. Being appreciative of people does help both them and us. At times we are all in an impossible situation that nobody would choose. However, I know I need to take responsibility for my reaction to everything. I learnt early on that other people, situations or things do not make you feel or do anything – you make that choice. Your reaction to anything is always yours to choose.

I could continue to feel anger, resentment and all manner of things. But I chose, for the sake of my own mental health and well-being, not to carry those feelings.

"Be kind whenever possible. It is always possible."

Dalai Lama

FOUR

Flapping About

Flapping is a huge help for Tommy which supports him to regulate himself. He does it with slinkies, socks, dressing gown cords: whatever he can get his hands on really. This stimming behaviour is a repetitive motion that he does with his hands that allows him to self-regulate sensory input. It keeps him in a calm state, like a comforter. Jumping on the trampoline does the same.

With a sensory processing disorder, he finds it difficult to process all the sensory inputs we are subjected to every day. The noises, smells, temperature changes etc that occur around us all the time. We have learnt to automatically turn down certain noises so they are just in the background. For Tommy every sense gets its input with the dial turned up to the max. It's like a constant attack on the system and without the capability to process those inputs instantaneously like the majority of us can without even thinking. He can end up in overwhelm with an overload of noise, smell or sight to deal with manually. This can lead to meltdowns, but flapping and stimming help him with this and often averts him from escalating.

However, flapping anything and everything did cause some stares when in public.

Out in Public

My flapping was something different. I began to find it harder to take things in my stride and would stress about everything- mostly down to what other people would think about me and how they would perceive us. In the early years when out and about with Tommy I found the general reaction from the public upsetting at times. He didn't look any different to any other toddler, but his behaviours did get some looks, comments and at times some direct feedback to my face. Using cutlery to eat his food was always challenging for him so he used his fingers a lot. That also created a mess around him and on the floor. He loved touching things in the shops, and at garden centres he liked to pull the flower heads off the plants.

In cafés when he saw something on someone's plate that he wanted he would just try and pinch it from them.

At first, my reaction was apologetic to anyone who was near. Trying to discipline him to behave like other toddlers that would understand what you were saying and why, was just not going to work. We avoided certain places. However, we did need to go shopping, eat out and do normal things other families did. My apologies turned to trying to explain to people, but it was impossible in just a few words.

Being out and about with Tommy has taught me a lot. He has no filter and knows nothing of social norms. As a young child, he was a cute, gorgeous-looking boy with blonde hair and curls. He turned heads with his smile. People tend to forgive a lot of what children do when they do things unexpected or different, as most people are kind. Not everyone though. Tommy pushed boundaries and I learnt a lot about giving up embarrassment and being over-apologetic.

I started to relax and not get concerned about what other people thought. It's about perspective. When at one time the thought of being out in public without makeup on was unthinkable, today I am often without makeup due to many reasons. From not having time when getting everyone else out of the house in accordance with Tommy's time, to just not having the energy.

Perspective helps everything. We all have things that were so important to us at an earlier age that now we look back on and just smile as to how far we have come. Knowing more now we can see with perspective how those important things have moved down the priority scale in our life now.

I often think of the line in a Robbie Williams song, *Youth is Wasted on the Young*. Just think how different our younger years would be if we could go back with the wisdom we have now. So much just wouldn't matter and any stress and worry would be put into the perspective of today. It's not that I don't care anymore about what others think of me with no makeup on. I do want to present myself the best I can and it's part of my self-care to feel good about myself. What I have given up is the comparison of myself with others. It helps absolutely no one.

It's Just Poo

When he was around five or six I took him to an out-of-town department outlet. He was still in nappies at this point; he wandered around holding my hand trying to touch everything in sight. We never stayed long in any one place as he always wanted to let go of my hand and run everywhere. So it was a short visit; get in, pick up what I wanted and head to the checkout. My sister was with me at the time as I always needed some help with him when outside. At the checkout queue I was holding his hand to my right, with my left I got out my purse and I noticed the checkout lady looking at him with astonishment. I turned around; he had dug deep into his nappy with his other hand and was smearing it all over his face as he really enjoyed the sensory feel of it. I reacted calmly and asked my sister to take him to the toilets which were close by. I turned back, paid for my items and said, "It's just poo," and joined my sister to clean him up.

I'm sure many other shoppers that day had a story to go home and tell. As a cute young boy, he could get away with a lot, but what about now as an eighteen-year-old man - tall, bearded, well built? Would he get the same reaction from the public if he did that now? There is still every possibility that he would do it again out in public, as he still enjoys the sensory stimulation it gives him and he has no awareness that poo on the face isn't a done thing. How would others react now?

This is his vulnerability and the reason for his carers to keep him safe. You never really know how anyone will react to someone they see behaving in a way they deem to be inappropriate.

Giving up on embarrassment is essential for this life. I re-framed it as educating the public on severe autism.

Another time we were at his favourite chip shop on the seafront in Penarth, seated outside with his sausage and chips. He enjoyed them as he always has. As he finished I could see he wanted to get up and go, which was never unusual as when he had finished his food and drink there was nothing else to hang around for, even if we hadn't yet finished eating. We learnt early on to either not have food with him, or get something that could be eaten quickly or taken away. As he got up I followed and he was heading back to the chip shop. Then he made himself sick right in front of the shop and all over the pavement where others were eating outside. He was going through this phase of making himself sick for some reason. The staff helped us with buckets of water to clean down the pavement, while I had to stop him somehow from going back into the shop. He had emptied his tummy of his food so he could have some more. Can't fault his logic there.

There are many similar stories of being out and about with him. In the beginning, I got hurt by the comments from others, sometimes made at me directly and some just uttered closely so I could hear. He loves sitting in cafes, eating his food, and always making a huge mess around him. The comments have reduced, or maybe I just don't have my radar on any more to hear them. They pass me by and if anyone does say anything I just smile at them with love. It helps with my own well-being to do that rather than get angry or upset with them and find some clever thing to say back. I let it go and don't hold on to that energy.

Meltdowns

He was becoming a teenager. His body was developing as teenagers do, he was growing taller and soon overtook me in height (not that difficult as I am only 4' 11"). His body was also getting stronger and we described him as not looking out of place in the rugby team front row. This started becoming difficult for me as he would use his whole body weight to move me into the places he wanted me to be. He has no sense of his body or his strength and would often sit on my lap as he used to, or put his whole body on top for a cuddle as he had done when younger. It was a dead weight as he had no concept of how it would feel for me.

Then puberty. From around the age of twelve, I was told that it was puberty that was the cause of his challenging behaviour. Was it? I really don't know and nor did anyone else. What causes someone to bang their head so hard into a concrete wall and develop an egg-like bulge on his forehead from so much head banging, that he still has to this day? What triggers him to escalate in an instant from calm and happy to hit out, especially at me, by tearing the skin off my arms or thumping me so hard in the chest I can't breathe? What I do know is that it isn't typical aggression from someone who is angry about something. A meltdown is what it means; a sudden and complete failure of something, in this case, his ability to control his body and behaviour as a result of something that has taken him to that melting point. It is NOT a conscious tantrum, nor a fight or flight response. It is an unconscious and inescapable escalation of being overwhelmed resulting in aggressive behaviour that he cannot control. This is just as frightening for him as it is for us.

As he developed further in his teenage years these meltdowns were getting more frequent, occurring multiple times a week. It was heartbreaking every single time. Seeing him like that for twenty or thirty minutes at a time self-harming and hurting me was hard. I was told to go somewhere else but I just wanted to help him, comfort him, make it stop. That's why I put myself in harm's way many times because if I could give just a little bit of comfort or help, then I didn't mind the scratches. I knew he didn't mean to hurt me; because once he had come back down and de-escalated, he wanted me to cuddle. I often asked him what did it feel like but he was unable to communicate. I wish I knew what was going on for him at those times.

When you feel helpless to change the horrible things in life for someone you love so much- what do you do? He didn't deserve a life that has been so hard for him. How as a parent do you make that better?

Cost of It All

For me, I just wanted to buy him things or give him food. At least I could help make him happy that way - I thought. If he showed just any interest in something I would try to get more of it for him. We bought him whatever I thought would make him happy.

He had the whole *Thomas The Tank* system of wooden tracks and engines as he loved watching the DVDs. I particularly liked the *Tidmouth Sheds* piece which was a huge wooden building with individual sheds for the engines, each having a track that led to a turntable in front. We built tracks for him going from room to room with loads of different unusual add-ons like the Quarry Shute or suspension bridge. He didn't play with it really. Having to push an engine didn't seem to be much fun, so, we bought the battery ones that just went around the track on their own. Again, just watching it didn't do much for him. I don't really think he made the association between the characters in the DVD and the toys.

We tried all sorts of different toys for all different ages to see if he would engage with any of them. Sometimes he did for a few minutes, like the ball drop, but soon got bored and didn't want to play with it again. He didn't really 'do playing' at all. I've never seen him actually pick up anything and go play with it. What he did like was interaction with adults. Never other children.

Financially it costs to have children. All the things they need as a baby, the toys as they grow up and everything else they want and need until they are adults. The money we paid out for Tommy was similar to all children in a lot of ways, but also different. As his body grew; his developmental age did not. He needed specialist nappies for young children, larger type buggies to keep him safe when we were out and a number of different items that were specialist, therefore expensive.

iPads have been our biggest spend, plus the gadget insurance we paid for each. Tommy goes through them quickly. Sometimes it can be months before one has its screen smashed, other times it's as if there is another one broken every week. We have tried all the cases and screen protectors possible to protect them but they still end up in tiny bits of glass and sometimes look like a banana. How he manages to bend them is beyond me. With the insurances we take out there is a constant cycle of iPads in use, being fixed or being written off and replaced. I often think we must be on a list somewhere and that one day John Lewis will prevent us from buying any more gadget insurance.

Shoes are another pricey item. He has very wide and very deep feet. He grew out of the normal wider-fitting shoes you can generally buy in his early teens. He now fits a 6E-8E(6V) shoe, which is the widest I have been able to find without needing them specifically made. These are really expensive and because he walks on the sides of his feet, they wear out quickly and need replacing every three months. He is currently seeing an orthotic consultant to try and help with the side walking.

Damage to the home that requires constant repairs. His strength allows him to pull doors from their hinges and make large holes in the plasterwork with his head. Even what would seem like a light, friendly punch broke TV screens.

Then there is the cost of hiring legal professionals to get the resources he needed from statutory services. The cost of having his SEN properly written by the Local Authority and the private assessments to go with it costs thousands.

In his later teens, his support needs were growing, and social services were not providing the level of support he needed. We had to cover this financially ourselves to ensure that he was safe out in public, his carers were safe and the public was protected too. There was a team of around six staff who we paid to take him out on a 2-1 basis after school and at weekends as social services deemed he only needed six hours of support a week.

All this meant that we were not able to give up work to get respite in the day while he was at school. We both worked full-time and provided care for him outside of school hours too. There was a huge financial pressure to just give us a kind of life that felt we could survive.

2:1 Support

We constantly asked for more support from social services. Others who were witnessing our life were also backing us up. I often drove him to school in tears and one such morning his social worker happened to be visiting his class and saw me. They were sympathetic and asked want we needed. I asked again for 24/7 care support at home. They just didn't have the resources, money or ability to provide what I was asking for.

Shortly after- as a strong, well-built, tall and bearded teenager - he was taken out to Barry Island for sausage and chips. He was only deemed by social services to need 1:1 support, meaning they assessed that he and others would be safe with just one other person with him. For months we had been asking them to provide 2:1 support. He was with Meg who had been his carer for a year or so in and out of school, after many others who had worked with him began to decline the work due to his growing strength. Meg was strong herself, inside and out, and had been able to handle him but she was also calling out for additional support when taking him out.

They were in the queue at the busy chip shop on the beach. He had queued there many times for his food and was anticipating it. He started to escalate and within seconds he had dragged Meg to the side by the low wall and managed to bite her deeply on her right boob. He wasn't letting go and in attempting to get him off he scratched her face causing blood to come from her face and her boob. There was no known trigger for this. Maybe he was overwhelmed by the anticipation of his food and was unable to process those emotions. When overwhelmed for any reason he erupts and is unable to handle or deal with what's going on in his body and goes into meltdown. An uncontrollable state.

Two lovely women came to help. They had observed that Tommy had special needs due to his demeanour and fortunately, they were both working as Learning

Support Assistants in a Special Needs School. Because of their experience and understanding, they knew what was going on. They were able to support Meg and Tommy as he began to de-escalate. They used her mobile to call me, got them safely to her car and stayed with them both until I arrived. I don't know who they were but if they ever read this book and recognise themselves, please get in touch as I would like to thank you. You were his earth angels that day.

It ended safely, but with Meg needing hospital attention. The scar on her face stayed with her. It could have been so very different though. Without being controlled Tommy would have run off and in that state who knows what damage he could have done to property or to others. Police may have gotten involved and again, without knowing Tommy could have made the situation worse by restraining him if they didn't know otherwise. Worse, the public witnessing this could have made the wrong assumption and seen - in their eyes - a man attacking a woman. It easily could have turned into something nasty.

He needs protection and the public need protection. He was assessed as needing 2:1 support after that incident, but it took that incident to push them to that decision. It absolutely should not have done. His need for 2:1 had been clear and well-articulated and argued for a while.

All Too Much

He continued to grow bigger and stronger. From an early age, I used food as a stress comforter and as a parent, I unconsciously tried to make him happy using food. This was a huge mistake as what started as something that would mean an interaction between us got out of hand. I would enjoy getting him a cake or biscuit as it made him happy. It was also a good way to develop some communication skills in terms of requesting it, in his own way, thereby reinforcing the concept of communication to ask for things.

Food became a huge motivator for him and it was used to motivate him to do many things. He even started saying some words again like Cake, Toast, and Biscuit, but not always in context. When he learned that a word got him something, then he used that word for everything he wanted. He developed a repertoire of a handful of words also including Slinky, Bus and Out. He learned from us that saying these things helped him express his desires. However, he used them for all things, at times when we weren't understanding what he really wanted as he just said them all in the hope one of them was right. One of them probably was, but we didn't know which.

One word though that always heals my heart is Jelly. I tell him often that "I love you lots like Jelly Tots" and one day he responded by saying the word Jelly. For me, this means he loves me too. Whenever I see him now and it comes to say goodbye, I always say, "Love you lots" and he says "Jelly". It melts me. Then as he drives off with his carers I still cry, and I'm good with that.

The connection between food and my presence got out of control. Whenever he was home and the carers had left, he would want me to take him out for a drive in the car. On this drive, he wanted a 'drive-through', whether chips, cake, biscuit or ice cream. I never knew which he wanted each time so ended up buying multiple things in the hope he wanted one of them, it was never the same every time. This ended up with him eating far too much and putting on weight, and me, eating what he didn't want at that time and also putting on weight. If I dared to drive past a usual place we visited I would get some behaviour from the back of the car which meant I had to turn around.

When we returned home after an hour or so of driving around, he went and chilled in his room. Sometimes for an hour or so, but sometimes just a few minutes before the demands to go out again started. Even if he had gone to sleep, if he woke in the middle of the night we had to go for a drive again.

Was I just giving in to him all the time? Yes, I was. I can hear the thoughts in your mind now as you read this. By giving in all the time was I just making it worse? Yes, I was. It came to the point that I would do anything, absolutely anything that he demanded so as not to get hurt either physically or emotionally. My nervous system was broken and it was the only thing I could do. I didn't have the strength to do anything different. I was in a state of constant stress. The agitation and anxiety caused me again to flap at the smallest thing that happened, and I just gave in.

I could see what was happening and I felt numb and unable to function properly. I reached out to friends who knew me well and had been looking out for me during this time. With the support of close friends around me, I was reminded to give as much time as I could to me; to my health and mental well-being. I took time off from work and spent the time Tommy was in school on sleep, rest or being outdoors. It was as much as I could manage.

It took a great deal of self-care to rebalance myself again, but in that short time, I was able to raise my consciousness again and attract different energies to me. This is such an important part of my life and what I coach. I know beyond doubt that a higher consciousness will result in better outcomes; with a greater feeling of hope that things will work out, then when things do start to get even a little bit better it becomes more self-fulfilling. But I often have to be reminded of this.

FIVE

Who Cares

The last eighteen years have certainly given us a new perspective on who stays around in your life and who runs a mile. I understand that your world changes completely when you have a family, it changes so much more when you are dealing with special needs.

"People come into your life for a reason, a season or a lifetime. When you figure out which one it is, you will know what to do for each person."

Friendships

It is inevitable that your circle of friends will consistently change during your lifetime and during the key phases of life, especially when children come along. Some you believe will stick around, don't, and others stay close regardless. The same with family. When you have a child who is different, with special needs or a disability, it felt to us like very few wanted to stay close. I do understand that happens and there is no malice here; my point is that the time you really need a circle of friends around you, there are very few that stay.

But there are new ones made too. The connection you crave with others facing similar challenges leads you to find new friends. In my case all with children with the same diagnosis. It was a relief to find out you were not alone. It seemed the more I looked, the more I found that the number of children with autism was much more than I thought, and it has seemed to grow exponentially over the years.

I joined a few parent groups and met some amazing people over the last eighteen years, all with challenges of their own within their families. All with help, advice and support to give. Friends that needed the most support were those who also readily gave their support. I hope some of these are lifetime friends, rather than seasonal ones. Time will tell, and whatever happens, will be good.

Over the years I also had support from a close circle of friends that I met when I began coaching when Tommy was very young; before I set up the charity. Although they didn't have the same life challenges as me, everyone has their own journey and challenges to face. What I found within this group were like-hearted people who provided support on an emotional level and helped with practical things, but most of all they listened, and heard me. Telling my story to people who I knew would not judge me, would provide a safe place for me to open up, and tell it how it is without the need to try and fix anything. To just listen and feel with me, hear me and validate all my feelings, thoughts and emotions has been one of the best gifts in my life.

As a coach, I have had a lot of training including NLP (Neuro-Linguistic Programming) and BC (Broadband Consciousness) which, for me, have remained the most powerful of all life skills. Even with these skills, a community of like-hearted and like-spirited friends is the essence of living. As humans we are meant to be connected - to help and support each other. It's not a race or a competition as to who can go faster, earn higher, get more qualifications or whatever comparisons you make with other people. The narrative we are given from a young age is naturally from those around us; our parents, carers, teachers and influential community members. Our script is written from their beliefs and values, not our own. As such we are not that person, even though we believe we are.

Marriage

The best friendship I have now is with my husband Alun. It has not always been like this and in the most challenging of times, we really had to hold on tight to what little we had left to give each other and avoid becoming another divorce statistic of parents with disabled children. Current statistics show that 80% of marriages that have a child with autism will end in divorce. This doesn't even include the people that stay in miserable marriages out of necessity. Up to 87% end in divorce if the child has disabilities. The figure is a lot higher when dealing with profound and multiple learning disabilities (PMLD), which can reach 95%. Thankfully we are not contributors to these statistics.

We held on. We always said we were a team, however, that really got tested on many occasions as we didn't agree on a lot when it came to Tommy.

Tommy's physical aggression towards me when he needed something he couldn't communicate, or was in pain or any emotional state really hurt us both. Alun hated the way he did that to me, and constantly asked me to get out of the room or lock myself away. I couldn't do it. He needed me and even though it was painful to watch him self-harm, or be the recipient of his behaviour, all I wanted to do was hug him and make it all go away for him. To have made myself absent at these times would have been, I believe, devastating for Tommy. I know Alun found it extremely hard to watch it and just wanted to protect me, but I wanted to stay and be there for Tommy.

When we were in the home together it was tense. Constantly waiting for the next thing that would happen. We were always on alert every minute with our ears picking up every little noise that came from wherever Tommy was, thinking is that a good noise or a bad one? Alun and I argued about all sorts of things and were very scratchy with each other. Yet, when we had the chance to get away, just for a meal or overnight sometimes, we reverted back to how we were when it was just us two. These moments were our respite and we valued them dearly.

Self-Care

At times over the past eighteen years, it felt like I was just about to drown. Keeping my face above water was all I could focus on. As long as I could still breathe I knew I would be okay. The increase in Tommy's challenging behaviour: the constant requests for help from social services and health teams, the incidents that were occurring due to a lack of support; the fear of him being in pain every time he cried out, the daily physical attacks and cuts on my body and the constant trauma putting my body into a constant state of imminent attack every time we were together took its toll.

In one particular MDT (Multi-Disciplinary Team) meeting, I cried all the way through. I was crying most of the time and couldn't, didn't want to, hold my emotions in. I had the empathy of all on the call, yet at the end of it, there was no further help available. I came off that call and felt completely broken. Let down with no end in sight. I honestly didn't know how I would manage to make it to bedtime. I spoke to my GP and was given anti-depressants. They weren't going to solve the issues but I had nothing else to try. After a while it did begin to feel that my head was above water and breathing was easier. Just with that small bit of help and in some moments of clarity of mind I was able to reach out to some close friends.

I was broken and unable to function. I had the responsibilities of a charity to manage with a team of staff that relied on me. I had Tommy to care for and look after, constantly driving him around day and night, a home to keep and it seemed that last on the list was me.

'Self Care Is My Super Power'. This is the mantra of an amazing group of women that I connect with regularly. The narrative we've been told all along as women are to put others first. Care for others before you consider yourself. This is a dangerous game to play and it can end up being the last straw for many men and women who cannot do any more for anyone as they have not taken care of themselves first.

You have to put yourself first, take care of yourself in order to be able to care for others. This is not being selfish. This is being the best you can be for you, therefore your family, loved ones and friends. If you don't do this, those that rely on your care will not get the best from you and you'll end up running on empty.

That's no good for you or anyone else. I live by this now and I know how different it feels to when I used to give all of myself to others first.

However hard it is to read this, please believe me it's the biggest truth of all. Self-care is your number one priority. I learnt this the hard way over the last eighteen years by giving more than I had to give.

Physically my body my back, neck and spine suffered. There were times when I just couldn't move off the bed or sofa, yet when Tommy wanted me to get up all the explanations in the world as to why I couldn't didn't matter. He pulled me up as he wanted something and I just had to do my best to move and get it for him. My skin also suffered particularly my arms. The frequent hitting and scratching took its toll. They were often red and raw from wounds upon wounds.

The emotional roller-coaster daily, even hourly was exhausting. Burnt out, broken, traumatised, a nervous breakdown together with high blood pressure is not a good place to be when you know you are still the main carer and responsible one. It was the day I acknowledged and accepted it that I was able to reach out and get some help.

Having frequent therapies for myself also helped a lot. It's not always accessible I know, but I believe that these sessions got me through it all. Osteopathy, acupuncture, massage and reflexology are my go-to treatments for renewal, energy and peace. On top of that though was the food and alcohol that also became my go too for helping to cope with each day. Not healthy, but I wasn't going to start beating myself up about it and kept it in some sort of control. Rekindled friendships with like-hearted people that cared and daily support online from my BC friends kept my energy in a better place. All that with the anti-depressants was my personal strategy for arriving at this point still in one piece.

Unconditional love for Tommy is one thing that I have and always will have. I am thankful daily for the experience of how this feels and what it means to give love unconditionally. Sometimes it feels glorious and sometimes it hurts so much, yet it's a huge positive from the whole experience that I am truly grateful to have received.

However, unconditional love isn't being a martyr to someone and sacrificing yourself for others. It can, and does, co-exist beautifully with self-care. It takes practice and it takes friends to keep reminding you.

SIX

Autistic Minds (The Charity)

It took time in the early years with Tommy to find my feet and navigate the whole support system of health, education, social services, therapies and even politics. During that time I kept a spreadsheet of people I connected with, services I found, websites that helped and all manner of information that was helpful. I joined advisory groups and later was invited to be part of the committee at the Welsh Government for the Autism Strategic Action Plan.

In 2010 I was having a cuppa at our local Ikea in Cardiff Bay and had the idea of a directory to share all the information I had collected and learnt about, the people who can help and how to contact them, the resources out there that were useful and some key information that I wished I had access to four years earlier. No one should feel alone on this journey. So I launched a company and website called The Autism Directory. You Are Not Alone.

It was a really basic website back then, but I kept adding information and resources to it as I researched and came across them. I built up a large number of 'friends' on Facebook and asked for help from others across the UK to help me populate it with more local information from different areas. It started to grow and the following year I applied for charity registration.

Over the following years, I continued to spend whatever time I could to keep it updated. However, other things in life took over my focus and so there were times when it didn't go anywhere. I managed to get a small team together to help out with marketing and website upkeep and from there it started to grow again. We had some funding help and rented a small office and hired staff. We started to diversify and launched training services and hired autistic staff to help. All of a sudden we were a constantly growing team adding more services and making an impact in the autism and autistic community.

As with all charities, funding is key and we relied so much on our community fundraising. When the pandemic hit in 2020 we lost that key income stream. We were able to apply for grants and managed to keep going with staff working from home, but it was a difficult time for all. Post-pandemic we were able to pick up and carry on with a different way of working and funding.

Now in 2023, we are called Autistic Minds. The Power Of Potential. Our name change reflected our broader range of services and the identity of our team. With just under fifty staff, 80% are autistic adults whom the charity has provided with employment opportunities.

You can find out more of what we do as a charity at www.autisticminds.org.uk, from help and community hubs, the autism directory (now at over thirty-two thousand entries), enterprises such as Ambition Prints and Safe Shred Wales, Independent Living Skills and In Work Support programmes, and other training and support services. We also put on annual Autism Exhibition Shows in Cardiff and Llandudno, with the aim of adding more across the country.

There is so much more I could share about the charity and what it has achieved to support others in the past thirteen years. What it has done for me though is priceless. We truly care: have committed to providing support at the grassroots level in the community and not be another faceless charity organisation.

Through the most difficult of times, the charity has given me a sense of purpose. When there is a team that relies on you and people that need your support, you get on with it. The team is also a huge support for me. They give me an insight into their world which helps me to understand my own son. Having a work-life to distract me from a challenging home life, particularly in the last three years, was another lifesaver.

I love the neurodiversity of the team that I still work with. Their input on what we do to support others in the same community always reminds me that we all have different maps of the world. We all can see things differently and that really helps each other across the team, whether neurodiverse or neurotypical.

"When you change the way you look at things, the things you look at change"

Wayne Dyer

Different Perspective

Isn't this quote so true? But why do we resist changing the way we see things?

I have often thought about the reasons for the exponential growth of autism diagnosis. I don't mean that I am looking for a cause, but wondering what it is that we need to listen to, and be taught so we can grow as humankind.

Why do autistic people feel like they don't fit in? Maybe because we have evolved into a society that has got a bit off the tracks and they don't want to fit into something that doesn't feel right.

In my experience as a mum and charity founder; autistic traits include no judgement, being truthful, saying what they mean and being authentic in who they are, how they show up and being true in all their communication. Being themselves and living in the moment. Accepting others for who they are and for what they stand for.

But we are raising our children and forcing them all to fit into our own map of the world - the one that generations before us have been doing. We don't seem to know any different. Values and beliefs are passed down to us and no one tells us how to discover our own. Our parents only project theirs onto us as if they were the right ones to have.

What if they are no longer willing to play that game? They are unique in themselves with their own ways of existing, thinking and communicating. Are we still not listening; intent on placing them in a box with a label that says they are different, not typical? Different for not fitting into a world that feels so wrong?

We judge and bring others down to make us feel good about ourselves. We look for things to make us feel better and crave that external validation from others. We are jealous because we are not comfortable with ourselves and our thoughts. Our society is full of blame - lying, cheating and harming others. There is fighting and killing. We no longer know who we are or why we are here.

They don't fit in because they can clearly see it is not something they want to fit into. They don't get it because it doesn't make any sense. Our world does not make any sense anymore and we are the ones labelling them for not getting it, for not understanding the world we have created because it doesn't make sense.

Just my pondering.

SEVEN

The Next Chapter

As a mother and parent, the last thing you want to accept is that you are part of the cause of the unrest and almost toxic environment at home. I am not and never have been toxic to be around, yet, the daily environment at home had become so.

I am definitely not proud of this, it was never intentional. My focus was always to provide a huge amount of love and loving energy at home. And it was that all along up to a couple of years ago when the impact of the trauma we were living in hit us. I don't use the word 'trauma' lightly. I have never been a person that collects labels of ill-health to feel my significance, and I am very aware that trauma is a huge deal for so many people, in so many different ways.

From around 2020, it started to get more noticeable. He was fifteen and gaining more strength in his body which he used a lot to get what he wanted. The hospital appointments and general anaesthetics he needed to remove the object up his nose, and the dental surgery fixing the exposed raw nerves. The beginning of his intense behaviour (not surprising with that tooth pain), but having to go through psychology and psychiatry assessments and trying different medications to calm him before the last resort of a general anaesthetic to discover the real issue. Covid certainly didn't help either in getting seen by professionals. My arms which had been scarred before from his meltdowns now were raw and covered with scratches and wounds on top of each other. The beginning of my nervous system learning to flinch every time I heard him stir in bed, wake up, walk around the house, or come near to me, not knowing what I was going to get. A lovely hug and kiss, or hurt by a hit and scratch that cut the skin. He was strong and used the full force of his body when he hit out.

That year broke me. I began to break down in my body and in my mental health. Every single day for three years we lived through this daily trauma which wasn't good for any of us. It developed slowly and unnoticeable for a while until we saw what we had become and what environment we had created at home. It wasn't good.

I say 'we' as both Alun and I went through this - but in different ways. Tommy always came to me and didn't want any interaction with his dad. When he hurt me, my husband was hurt too as he could see what state I was in and how I reacted emotionally. I don't think there was a day I didn't cry. We lived each moment expecting Armageddon, and at night too.

This energy throughout the home was toxic in the end. Tommy wanted to get out of the house at every opportunity and when he wanted me to take him for a drive - believe me when I say I didn't have any choice. Whatever time of the evening, night or day he would put his shoes on and say "car", take me to the front door, pick up my handbag (a point of reference to say he wanted to go out), and we would go for a drive. In the middle of the night if he woke up I knew that we'd be driving around for the next few hours. It really wasn't safe for me to drive alone with him as he could kick out at any time, pull my hair or take off his seatbelt and mine while we were moving. I had to stick to roads that I knew I could stop safely if needed, although that wasn't always possible.

Many times I had to stop and pull over, park up and get out of the car quickly while he had a meltdown in the back. I couldn't let him out of the car as he would just run away, so I had to keep him safe, locked in while I stood outside until he had managed to calm down again. One time I was driving through a village in the Vale and had to stop in front of some houses. I got out and he was banging the car so loudly on the windows that residents came out to see what was going on. I had to explain while sobbing why he was banging the car. I also had to really encourage one person not to call the police. Most people are nice. Few are not.

The self-perpetuating environment was not helping but we had no mental capacity to change. He was just reacting to the daily negative energy we were all creating. Not our fault nor his. We needed support as a family. Our friends helped as much as they could. Counselling sessions helped as much as they could. But our nervous system was shot to pieces a long while ago and in that place, we were physically, emotionally, and mentally unable to change the dynamic.

We asked social services many times what would happen if the worst were to happen to us. We were already in crisis and they recognised that, but still, no further support was provided. They said if we felt we needed to we would have to call the police. They would take him and find someplace for him. As if we were going to let that happen and it took every single cell in my body, every single ounce of energy to make it through each day so it didn't come to that. We were in crisis, in survival mode. All this created a really unhealthy place for Tommy and for us. Those weeks and months were awful. In fact, there isn't a word I could use to describe the hell we were all living in.

The Hardest Decision

Knowing that home was not the best place for him, I really struggled with the decision for him to move out to a home where the staff would look after him. They wouldn't love him unconditionally as I do. In the end, those 'best interests' meetings helped me to make that decision. In my head, I knew we all needed this. My heart felt broken again.

After Tommy's seventeenth birthday, the transition planning began. This was the transition from children's social services to adults. A completely new team that was going to have discussions with me about the rest of his life. All along I had been asking about what options there were for his long-term care. My desire was that we could somehow keep him home with a team of carers living in to provide the 24/7 care he needed. I had planned the house out and how that could work. However, this option was never entertained. I feared that the use of the term "best interests" would be used against me and what I wanted for him.

After more months of continued meetings leaving me feeling completely broken, the challenges continuing and getting more frequent at home, I broke. I threw in the towel - so to speak - and I asked for help in getting a residential placement for him. It had become an unrecoverable situation at home and we were not in a good place.

He was still seventeen at this point however adult services did start looking for somewhere suitable. It was as I had feared that nothing was looking available. It's not as if there is a turnover of residents in these care homes as there are with older people's care, which have frequent availability as their residents emigrate to heaven. Once the home was full, residents tend to stay for a very long time, especially if they go in as young adults.

A couple of places were found but they were not set up to be able to manage the challenging behaviours that Tommy had so they had to be discounted. Then a place that said they were able to meet his needs was found, but it was out of the county about an hour away from home. Not ideal, but I thought it was only an hour away and not many hours away. We went to visit and it ticked all the boxes we had. However, something didn't feel right and I couldn't put my finger on it. But it was the only option available. We didn't get the chance to view and compare with others, it was this or nothing.

My cognitive dissonance was going wild. I always said I would never allow him to go into a home run by a large company. Too many stories of abuse and many more stories not told. I started to look for the positives about the company and home and tried to make myself believe them. We had to move ahead and meetings and plans were made for him to move in. It was due to be as soon as possible and they said they could take him before he was eighteen, but it transpired they couldn't. Providing care for children is so much more regulated and although he was only a couple of months away from being an adult, it would not be possible as they didn't meet those regulations.

So a moving date was agreed as the day after he was eighteen. I spent time getting things for his room and moving things in. Then two weeks beforehand we had a call. They didn't have enough staff so it would have to be postponed for about a month so they could recruit. I initially felt devastated. Not that I wanted to get rid of him, but I had no more in me to carry on. That night, however, as I lay in bed I had the most overwhelming feeling of relief. It was so powerful that I committed to not letting him go there. It wasn't right for him and I knew it all along.

The next day we were back to square one and with his social services and health teams we had to reconsider. It was interesting that no one else disagreed with me when I said he didn't belong there and I wouldn't let him go. Another place had been found but this one was an hour and a half away towards West Wales. I had a look on their website and it was a small family business with only a small number of rooms. It gave me hope again. While looking into the company on the Care Commissioners website I discovered that they also had a home only half an hour away from us. I got excited. Researching further I then found that home up for sale. I felt gutted again.

We went ahead and arranged a meeting with the owner. Completely a different experience as she came out to our home and had a long conversation about what we wanted for Tommy. She listened and I felt she heard us too. I asked her about the house she had up for sale only half an hour away and she said she had taken it off the market and was going to open it back up as a residential home, that Tommy could be the first resident. This was great news.

It was going to take some time to do up the house and recruit staff but she confirmed end of January 2023 was a possible moving date. This wasn't too far away and with renewed optimism, I knew we could make it till then and wait for this date so he could go there.

His eighteenth birthday came along and because he was meant to have been in the first home by then, there was no provision available to support him at home. So agency staff were commissioned to help us temporarily. We were grateful for the help, but the staff, in the majority, were hard to work with as they really didn't understand Tommy. Again we were told these staff had experience with autism. Great, but do they have experience with Tommy's autism? It's that one diagnosis that covers so many different presentations that I knew they didn't have a clue. One person left within half an hour, and another looked so frightened we said she could go. Most didn't sign up for a second session with him. There were a few exceptions and these few ended up supporting him on rota between them.

Christmas came and went and we were in January 2023. The new faces coming in all the time and the tension that we all felt in the house was hard. The staff covered after school until about 9 pm and on weekends from 9 am to 9 pm. The hours outside that were still down to us at home. Whether it was the energy at home or not that made Tommy want to be out all the time I don't know, but, all he wanted was for me to take him in the car for a drive. If he was awake he wanted to be out. By this time I had nothing left in me to do anything but comply. I just surrendered and whatever the time, if he woke we went for a drive. He was due to be dropped off at school at 9 am, so we would often go out hours before that and drive around until it was time for school.

The date for moving into the new home was looming again and another call informed me of a delay by another four weeks so staff had time for proper training on Tommy's needs. Totally understandable and I wouldn't have wanted him to move in with them not having that. Nonetheless, it was another devastating blow.

Another delay. Another month.

A Brick Wall

One morning I was preparing to take Tommy to school. I remember the day as it was Alun's birthday. After the drive during the night, it was raining when we got back so I parked the car closer to the house than usual. This meant in the morning I had to move the car slightly for Tommy to be able to get in. He was out in the driveway with me looking for his slinkies in the drive that he regularly chucked there from the garden. I jumped in the driver's seat - looking to move it just a metre forward and slightly right. I put my foot on the accelerator to gently move forward, but instead, my foot pressed the pedal hard and I darted ahead, through our fence and into the neighbour's house wall. In slow motion, I can re-live it now. I had lost the ability or capacity to know how to put my foot on the brake. Instead of gently moving, I had floored the pedal and shot off. It was only about five metres but enough to break through the fence at the top of our drive, crash into next door's house and concertina the engine into half its size.

Our property is elevated at the top of the drive, with our neighbour's property about fifteen feet lower than ours. I had no seat belt on, and I hadn't closed the car door. I was only meant to move it about a metre. As the car crashed into the wall it tilted to the right and was being held up by the back wheels still on our drive and the front firmly planted in the house walls. My door was open, no seat belt and on a right tilt with a fifteen-foot drop below me. I watched the front of the car against the walls and begged it not to move. I tried to ascertain if this was real life or a dream. It was happening in real life.

So I breathed and remained calm and very still. A voice behind me asked if I was okay. I said yes but I need help. Alun came out, saw the situation and called 999. I waited for what felt like an age, not daring to move and my muscles tight to keep me in position, all the while watching the car didn't start to slide down the wall. I actually considered whether this would be the end of me if the car did suddenly drop. I felt strangely calm. Then I began to shake.

Within five minutes I had three fire engines, an ambulance and two police cars arrive. The emergency services were amazing. They talked to me explaining every step of what they were going to do. They secured the rear of the car and then with weight pulling down on the left side I was to pull my seat back and climb onto the back seat. I couldn't reach the lever for the seat to move so one of them reached over from where the fence should be and moved it back. I climbed to the back seat and then was helped out.

Paramedics checked me over and did some tests including blood pressure. Naturally, this was high at the time but they said it would come down over the next half hour. Two hours later sat in the ambulance it was still high. I wonder whether I would have ever found out otherwise that I needed treatment for ongoing high blood pressure.

The school was called to come and get Tommy and he saw me in the ambulance as they drove past. I have no idea what he was thinking or if he knew what was going on. It must have impacted him somehow. He did witness the crash but was taken inside soon after. The police were happy that there was no crime and eventually everyone left.

I sat in the house wondering what had happened. Trying to relive those moments to figure out what I did. All I can remember is my foot on the accelerator and not being capable of taking it off or using the brake. I cried a lot and eventually sent a message to close friends to tell them what had happened and ask if anyone had a sofa. I needed to leave home if I was going to survive. I knew I couldn't do another hour at home - Tommy was due back at 3 pm.

This is when you get to find out who cares. Meg, now a close friend and carer for Tommy drove over to the house, helped me pack a bag and took me back to hers to stay. Tommy still needed a carer so she left her husband, Simon, at the house in exchange to stay with Tommy and do all the things that I usually did for him. It was meant to be a short respite stay but I ended up living with her for six weeks - and Simon with Tommy and Alun. At that time social services, health and the new residential care provision agreed on a move-in date for him. Meg also took over from me being the main contact in terms of his transition into his new home.

I just needed to sleep, be cared for myself and begin my journey of recovery. Meg and Simon, whom we now call family, were there for me, Tommy and Alun in every way.

I couldn't go on and the Universe stepped in. The car crash was the best thing that happened to me. I hit a brick wall - literally - emotionally and physically and surrendered to being cared for.

As much as that respite was needed, I felt so much guilt in being away from Tommy. We met at least weekly outside of the home for an hour or so, with me learning how to be his mum, not his carer. When it was time for him to get back in his car and say goodbye, it was so emotionally tough. I hated that no one could explain to him what was happening; that mummy wouldn't be coming home again and that soon he would have another place to live.

Moving Out

Those six weeks did turn out to help make his transition to his new home easier and more gentle. We got into a routine of meeting out, having something to eat and saying goodbye. It was winter so we were very limited on what we could do in the late afternoons. Then the day came for him to move.

It was decided in his 'best interests' for me not to be involved. He was taken out for the day by Meg and Simon and then after they drove to his new home. He had visited there twice before on tea visits so he was familiar, and he knew there was a bedroom with a TV and DVD player. He had his new suitcase with him. When he had been going to his respite place before, the suitcase was always an object of reference so he knew he was going somewhere. With his suitcase with him, I guess he knew he was going to stay over at the new place too.

Feeling so anxious, and still very guilty for him moving out and me not being with him was incredibly tough, however, I knew it was the best approach for him. The six weeks of transition and our separation really were a blessing. The communication was good with the staff at the new home. They emailed me each evening to tell me about his day and how he was feeling and behaving. He was being taken to school each morning by staff and picked up again, each afternoon, so that was also a stable and familiar routine for him.

By the first weekend, I was worried that he might be expecting to come home again soon. He only ever went to respite for a few nights and it had been 4 nights now. Managing his routine on a weekend was always a challenge and they got through it with little problem. The next week I was still getting reports of good days with some challenging moments, but nothing like the behaviour we had seen at home.

After a few weeks it was Easter Holidays, and the first time he would be there without the routine of school for two weeks. They all found this especially hard as he needed his daily routine to keep him calm and regulated. It was a new experience for him, and the staff, with some very challenging moments. An insight for them as to what they needed to think about for the upcoming summer school holidays.

Thoughts From Dad

I offered Alun a part in this book. This is what he wanted to say.

The biggest lesson in hindsight was coming to understand Tommy's challenges with anxiety. Understandably most look at other people's anxiety in terms of their own perceptions and experience so we often needed to dig deep to really understand his. The triggers are different for everyone, so coming to understand his was a huge learning experience and an awakening.

A lot of what we had to do was manage the manifestations of his anxiety without knowing anything about it. The fact that he could not manage that process verbally meant we were always scrabbling in the unknown. Stumbling about in the dark. This realisation came much later than would have liked.

I sneezed and he would have a go at me. If my sneezing caused his anxiety then it's not to be trifled in any way. It's different for everyone. I believe that in general our society treating children like shit is normalised, their anxieties and emotions are either not properly taken into account or are trivialised.

I generally felt really upset and frustrated. Severely traumatised and permanently braced for an apocalypse due to living with someone with limited ways of expressing his frustration and anxiety. All he did was to use the methods at his disposal and he had to develop these strategies himself for managing his life.

In his new place now he is different. His default position is no longer to go to the fridge – because they have worked hard with positive affirmations. At home, we were so battered – get punched or give him a slice of toast. I now have the emotional strength and energy to process other life stuff.

I got a bike out of the attic the other day. That may not sound like a big deal in any way, but for me, it was a big thing. I first bought the bike back in 2019 so that I could cycle to work from my digs. I was living and working in Milton Keynes at the time - commuting home by car at weekends - and wanted to get back into getting to and from work by bike during the week. Due to reasons, the bike never got unpacked, so it travelled back with me in its box when that work finished.

The bike remained in the attic for almost four years. A recent conversation with my manager eventually led me to unpack it, set it up and ride it around our yard. Sounds simple yet for me, it's about having the emotional space and energy to be able to not only do something like that but also to think about the possibilities and freedoms which it could afford me.

For so long much of my emotional budget and time was consumed by the trauma. Either waiting for an event, dealing with an event or recovering from an event. I've been running on fumes for so long now I don't know any other way. My household priorities have been just about getting through the basics; laundry, cooking and bins. Most other things I just couldn't even contemplate. I know that sounds odd and I get that you might not understand it, but for me it was real.

Stress and the processing of trauma manifest themselves differently in people. For me, my stomach and gut have always been my second brain. And I've always had a complex relationship with food, having been brought up with the script of "you will eat when we say, what we say and how much we decide to put on your plate". My relationship with food is far more amicable and healthy now, but I can still remember feeling rather hard-done-by in being described as a child who was fussy or picky with food. There is nothing wrong with a child expressing a preference.

My way of dealing with trauma was to be sick. For the past few years, I've been sick on a weekly basis, with no physical prompt; no reason such as overindulgence or illness behind it. I'm just glad that I've been able to realise that and grateful, as there are many worse ways in which one's body could process trauma.

On a positive note, living in the moment entirely is a special and unique lesson we learned from our son, Tommy.

EIGHT

An Adult Child

He is now an adult. A man. Also still developmentally a child.

What will his future look like? These are my constant thoughts and questions I ponder.

Does he get the concept of growing older; what life tends to pan out like with partners, work, kids and other opportunities that we strive for? Does he get all that and understand how difficult that might be for him? Or is he oblivious to it all?

In his world with no concept of this, what does he have to wake for each day? We all deserve to have something in our lives that gets us out of bed and maybe for him that's simply to go out for a drive in the car and watch *Bob The Builder* on his iPad. Does it matter that there isn't something fulfilling him in his life? Is it just simply he is either happy or he is not? What determines that? Maybe he is simply happy when he gets what he wants; a slinky toy, cake or for someone to take him outdoors. Is it that simple? Is it us that overcomplicates happiness?

His life is lived without having goals or anything to aim for, even if just looking forward to a holiday. We are all told the narrative of striving for something, setting goals, and achieving them is all-important for our self-worth. What if it isn't? With goals comes the fear of failure, which isn't failure at all but that's what we are told in order to fear us into doing something. Is it a better way to live to just wake up and our default mode is to be happy, after all, we've won the biggest lottery of all when we do wake up to another day. Think about that. What would you choose – to win millions on the lottery or wake up the next day?

What emotions does he feel? Happy, sad, confused, upset, frustrated, angry. I'm sure he does feel these but how does he process them and what thoughts accompany them? Since being a baby he hasn't really cried at all. Do these emotions simply come and he just lets them go without the need for their physical expression, or do they stay in his body without being processed at all? That's both scary and upsetting to think.

What about love and sex? He is a fully grown man and although I know he's had time in his room alone, I don't know if it has ever come to anything. Maybe as his mother, I don't need to know that stuff; but it has been difficult to see him mature in his body and not his mind, go through adolescence and not be able to explain these things to him, not knowing what to do and not able to help. I discussed this with his health team and asked about professional health-led sex workers. They are a thing apparently, but it was never followed up.

His life will be taken care of by others. He is in a residential home now being looked after by a team of day and night staff. He has no work to go to and to get stressed about. No money issues to know about. He will get fed, clothed, taken out and will always have someone with him to look out and care for him. His personal hygiene is done by others; washing is done for him and has an endless stream of things to watch on his iPad. Sound good? Would you choose that life if it also meant having severe autism and profound multiple learning disabilities? Or would you take the life you have now with all the problems you perceive you have?

"Millions of people would love the life you have. Be one of them."

Richard Wilkins

Our responsibility to create a life for him so he always has enough money and is cared for by the right people so that he will never be put in a vulnerable situation, is emotionally tough. That's on top of the emotional challenges that we've been through so far - missing out on key celebrations and life experiences that we should have had as parents of a young boy.

On Mother's Day and Father's Day, his learning support assistants at school made some cards for us and had him do a handprint or splash some paint on it. Same with Christmas. These annual events were so very different for us as a family. He had no concept of them.

We never had the opportunity to take him to birthday parties; nor taxi him and his friends around for football club, swimming or whatever it would have been for him. He didn't engage with other children at school, only the adults, so never had friends that would come over.

In the summer of 2021, we should have been anticipating his GCSE results with him. Instead, I scrolled through social media seeing others celebrating their children's results while in the background *Bob The Builder* was on repeat, interrupted now and then with some *Teletubbies* or *Fireman Sam*.

At eighteen we should have bought him a car. A symbol of independence and becoming an adult. Instead, he had more slinkies and a replacement iPad for the ones that were smashed.

We have never been able to apply for a bank account for him as he couldn't sign his name and he didn't have the capacity to understand what he would be signing for. All his finances now as an adult have to go through a trust, managed by trustees.

Future Years

Looking forward now, we will have no daughter or son-in-law to know.
No weddings or ceremonies to celebrate.

No grandchildren to love and care for.

No work successes or life achievements to be proud of.

None of it is his fault and we are not blaming anyone for any of it.

We are just incredibly sad about it.

That was the bit in the Brochure we wanted.

He is now in residential care for the rest of his life. He is just eighteen and I can't get my head around that. When old people can't look after themselves, they go into residential care. Is it really the right place for my eighteen-year-old son? Maybe it's just the name 'residential care' that gives the connotations of old people sitting in the lounge all day and sleeping. He is active and wants to be outdoors all the time.

The emotional journey I had to go through to say yes to him moving to a place like this. The guilt of letting him go, leaving home one morning and not returning again without the opportunity to explain anything to him that he would understand. The terrors from all I have heard regarding places that abuse the vulnerable kept me up at night.

My fears are about whether they will care for him properly. Will they care about him as much as I do?

Will they put his socks on for him so the seams are straight and don't feel tight? His shoes too, ensuring the sole isn't crumpled under his feet and the Velcro straps are not too tight? Pants on properly and straight so as not to cause discomfort up the bum. Shorts or trousers are on properly and not skew-whiff or twisted at the waist. Pockets in smoothly and not crumpled up. All these things with clothing can cause discomfort but he wouldn't know himself how to correct them or make anyone aware.

But the most worrying thing of all is keeping an eye on his health and well-being. He cannot say or express when something is hurting. He may just become aggressive which can easily be misinterpreted. Missing out on the usual signs of something not being right health-wise is a major concern.

Will he miss going on holiday? He doesn't have the concept of the world, or that there are different countries and places to go and see. As a young boy, we did take him on a few holidays. In reality that was our 'map of the world' in that we thought it would make him happy to go abroad. We took him on a plane as a baby to Spain; on Eurostar to Brussels, on cruises to Venice and Baltics. As a young child, it was easier to manage, especially with a carer with us too. As he hit his teenage years this became more difficult. Being abroad scared me: if he did have a meltdown in public would they understand? Would they be less compassionate and aware - call the police if he started being aggressive? If he was taken ill, would the hospitals have the knowledge to deal with his severe autism? Would anyone really understand? It became too much of a risk and from then we stayed close to home. Close enough to be able to go home if needed and to the health and social worker teams who knew him.

Does he enjoy being away from what he knows as home? I'm not sure, I think so. It's a change for him and now we have found somewhere ideal for holidays where he knows, it's like another home from home for him which is familiar, safe and enjoyable. I guess only time will tell.

I have no idea what the future will be for him. He has another year in school and then… what? What will he be doing for the rest of his life? What will he be waking up and looking forward to? Whatever it is, I just hope it makes him happy.

NINE

Our New Journey

This book has been written in the months following when Tommy moved into residential care - at a point when we are both starting to recover from these last few years. This is now a new journey that we are excited about but it comes with a lot of guilt and sadness that it came to be too much for us and Tommy; the only option was for him to be in a place where teams of professional carers can look after him. It was the right decision for everyone, but that doesn't make it any less emotional.

A large part was written in Brussels on a weekend a couple of weeks after his move. The trip became a significant turning point from one life to another, and very symbolic in that it was the beginning of us allowing our healing to begin.

I had an email telling me we had some unused Avios points. Normally my reaction would have been to pass it by and do nothing as there was no way we could go away without a huge amount of planning to arrange childcare with the very few people that knew him well, people we could trust, and this came at a significant financial cost too. I was about to delete it as irrelevant and the realisation came over me 'What's stopping us'? We didn't have the childcare to think about, the trip would be paid for with points and we had the time.

The guilt of the situation took over me and it felt like running away from our own son. It caught me off-guard and the emotional waves flowed. I had learnt how to 'lean into' my feelings instead of pushing them away. To feel the emotions I have with intensity and allow them to be, to let them do what they need to and allow them to pass in their own time.

There is no fear in feeling one's feelings. We each have a huge range of them to help us with all aspects of our lives. We need to learn how to use them so they can do just that. However, we learn from a young age that there are positive feelings which are good to have, and negative feelings that we shouldn't have and these must be pushed down, stopped from arising and kept inside. This is so not the healthy thing to do. Feelings are neither positive or negative, they are what they are and come to us to help in various situations. What behaviour we then manifest with these feelings is another thing entirely, and this we can choose every time. Crucially, we have that choice.

Just because we are feeling angry doesn't mean we have the right to behave angrily with another person or property. Disassociating the feeling (I feel angry) from the identity (I am angry) that drives behaviour is our own responsibility. Also pushing the feelings away or keeping them inside is hugely unhealthy too. If they are not processed by feeling them, and with the intensity they require, they stay as unprocessed energy fields in the body that can become dis-eased, and we get unwell.

I can feel guilt and sadness without being guilty or sad and this is a huge distinction I can make every time now. So I booked the flights, hotel and travel and we were in Brussels that weekend. The sense of freedom was a great start on this new journey for all of us.

On our return, we left Heathrow and joined the M4 home. Then we had the realisation. This would be the first time that we would, as a married couple, be returning back to our home, and Tommy would not be there. This could have been a sense of loss and perhaps we had some feelings of 'empty-nest' syndrome. But that wasn't it.

We realised that we weren't feeling the anxiety or the stress as we had done every other time we snatched a weekend alone here and there. There would be no handover notes, no run-down about how the weekend had gone, and no report on any further damage to the house. We could just go home, pour a drink and put Netflix on. Like normal people.

To say that we felt privileged and thankful to be able to do this would be a huge understatement.

It's now only a few months since Tommy moved to his new home and we are just beginning to remember who we are again. It will take time, and we will have new ideas and opportunities to explore. One thing that doesn't change though is that I am still his mum. I see him weekly and we have lots of hugs and kisses. He is then happy to say bye-bye and Jelly.

Now I must finish that packing and I can't wait to see him later today in West Wales for our family holiday.

Final Thoughts

Build your village and ask for help. People want to help.

Avoid victim mode. Sometimes you fall into it but learn to recognise that's where you are and quickly reframe it. Find a strategy to move out of that mode. Write a gratitude list, refer to it often and keep updating it. You won't see the opportunities to improve the situation from a place of being a victim, they just won't be on your radar to notice. From a place of gratitude and whatever strength you have to see the possibilities you will find a way to increase your consciousness, and then miracles can happen.

Seek nature as much as possible. Open the windows daily if nothing else. Walk in parks, go near the water, and find some trees. Hug a tree and give it all your worries and emotions that you wish to let go of. It will process those energies and send them back into the earth to be alchemised.

Believe in things that you want to believe in, even if you can't find anything to base that belief on. Just choose to believe for no other reason than you want to. I believe when our soul leaves our body we just emigrate to a different place in the Universe. Energy cannot die it just transforms, therefore we cannot die. Do I need to look for the science in quantum physics to provide that? No, I just believe it because I don't want to believe an alternative. I may be wrong but my life is so much better with the beliefs I choose to have while I'm here.

Believe whatever you are going through now will get better. With that belief, you will see the opportunities to make it so. If you believe nothing ever goes right for you then you will continue to find those opportunities to prove your belief right. This alone is a powerful tool to change your life.

Your 'script' will always try to get you to focus on the negative. Your script is the negative voice in your head that tells you that you aren't enough, that life will always be tough or whatever else it uses to keep you from living fully. You will know your own particular script well and what it constantly wants to remind you of to keep you at a low consciousness. You may not be aware but that voice is not you. We are told that it is but believe me it is not.

Your script was handed down to you by your parents, carers, guardians and all other influential people in your past, maybe teachers or religious guides even. They got theirs from their ancestors and so it goes way back and can be very convincing to you that it's the truth. Your beliefs and values in the world are theirs, not yours. You can choose what you think and you don't need to have any thoughts that are no longer helpful. You don't need to listen to it. This is another book though!

I hope that something in our story has helped in some way. You can follow our page on Facebook and other socials. Search for the title of this book to find us. Thank you.